STRONG&
Sculpted

Brad Schoenfeld, PhD, CSCS, CSPS, FNSCA

HUMAN KINETICS

Library of Congress Cataloging-in-Publication Data

Names: Schoenfeld, Brad, 1962- author.
Title: Strong & sculpted / Brad Schoenfeld, PhD, CSCS, CSPS, FNSCA.
Other titles: Strong and sculpted
Description: Champaign, IL : Human Kinetics, [2016] | Includes
   bibliographical references and index.
Identifiers: LCCN 2015049352 | ISBN 9781492514565 (print)
Subjects: LCSH: Bodybuilding for women. | Physical fitness for women. |
   Weight training.
Classification: LCC GV546.6.W64 S36 2016 | DDC 613.7/045--dc23 LC record available at
http://lccn.loc.gov/2015049352

ISBN: 978-1-4925-1456-5 (print)

Acquisitions Editor: Michelle Maloney
Senior Managing Editor: Amy Stahl
Copyeditor: Patsy Fortney
Indexer: Dan Connolly
Senior Graphic Designers: Fred Starbird and Keri Evans
Cover Designer: Keith Blomberg
Photograph (cover): © AYakovlev/iStock.com
Photographs (interior): Neil Bernstein
Visual Production Assistant: Joyce Brumfield
Photo Production Manager: Jason Allen
Art Manager: Kelly Hendren
Associate Art Manager: Alan L. Wilborn
Illustrations: © Human Kinetics
Printer: Walsworth

We thank Premier Athletic Club in Montrose, New York, and The Refinery in Champaign, Illinois, for assistance in providing the locations for the photo shoot for this book.

Printed in the United States of America   10 9 8 7 6 5 4 3 2 1

The paper in this book was manufactured using responsible forestry methods.

Human Kinetics
Website: www.HumanKinetics.com

United States: Human Kinetics
P.O. Box 5076
Champaign, IL 61825-5076
800-747-4457
e-mail: info@hkusa.com

Canada: Human Kinetics
475 Devonshire Road Unit 100
Windsor, ON N8Y 2L5
800-465-7301 (in Canada only)
e-mail: info@hkcanada.com

Europe: Human Kinetics
107 Bradford Road
Stanningley
Leeds LS28 6AT, United Kingdom
+44 (0) 113 255 5665
e-mail: hk@hkeurope.com

Australia: Human Kinetics
57A Price Avenue
Lower Mitcham, South Australia 5062
08 8372 0999
e-mail: info@hkaustralia.com

New Zealand: Human Kinetics
P.O. Box 80
Mitcham Shopping Centre, South Australia 5062
0800 222 062
e-mail: info@hknewzealand.com

E6638

Foreword

My love affair with lifting weights started in high school with one of those home gyms. Nothing fancy, but adequate enough to get a decent workout. I started with a variety of exercises, seeing how much I could lift. When I tried the leg press, I found I could do the entire weight stack. That was a rush. I loved the sensation of pushing weight, taxing my body to its limit. I was hooked.

It wasn't until college that I really got serious about lifting. I attended the University of Florida on a track and field scholarship, where I competed in the high jump. The university had an amazing strength program and a state-of-the-art fitness center. My motivation to train was purely competition related. All I wanted was to increase strength and power to optimize my athletic performance; I really couldn't have cared less about the aesthetic aspect.

I gravitated to performing the Olympic lifts and powerlifting moves. Squats were a favorite; I started with the bar and worked my way up to 275 pounds (125 kg)—more than double my body weight.

I experienced great satisfaction in lifting as much weight as possible and seeing how it translated to my performance in the field. I got faster. I could jump higher. That motivated me to train even harder. I ended up earning Junior All-American status, which I attribute largely to my fitness regimen.

When I had been out of college for several years, I was still jumping, although no longer competitively. For fun, I began working out with the USA Track and Field team. With diligence and hard work, I was able to clear 5 feet 11 inches (180.3 cm) in the high jump—my all-time best. My coach said that if I could clear 6 feet (182.9 cm), I'd be able to participate in the Olympic trials.

I was focused. All my energies were channeled into eking out that extra inch (2.5 cm) in the high jump. I trained harder than ever. It never happened.

I was so discouraged. I'd worked so hard to accomplish my goal, and now all hope for an Olympic tryout was gone. I suddenly had nothing left to train for, no goal to serve as motivation.

Shortly thereafter, I was thumbing through a fitness magazine, and a friend suggested that I consider doing a figure competition. At first I dismissed the notion. I grew up as a tomboy, not a girly girl. The thought of parading around in a swimsuit wasn't all that appealing.

But without any other competitive aspirations at the time, I decided to give it a go. At the very least, it gave me something to train for.

I won the first competition I entered; my motivation soared. I entered another show and won again. Then I entered and won a national competition, at which I earned my pro card.

I placed 10th in my initial pro show—the 2009 Arnold Classic—and then took 6th at the 2009 Figure Olympia. After that, I never finished outside the top three. The highlight of my career came in 2010 when I won the pinnacle of women's physique competitions, the Figure Olympia—and then I did it again two years later!

When I tell my story, it sounds as though things came easily for me. Nothing could be further from the truth. Physique competition requires optimal shape and symmetry. I was lagging in both.

I'm a right-handed thrower and a right-footed high jumper. As a result of years of track and field work, my left side was seriously lagging over my right. Moreover, my calves were out of balance with my thighs, and I needed to bring up my glutes as well as improve my shoulders and lats.

I was able to overcome these obstacles because of an intense work ethic, an unending drive to succeed. Sure, I have good genetics. But so do millions of other women. To rise to the top requires dedication and hard work. There is no substitute. The good news is that these are qualities that everyone can develop.

If you're new to lifting, start out by learning the basics. Perform mostly compound movements involving the large-muscle groups. Build a strong base. Focus on proper form. Only after you have achieved these attributes should you begin to work on lagging areas and incorporate some of the literally hundreds of exercise variations into your routine.

One of the greatest challenges is to be patient and set objective and realistic goals. Understand that developing a terrific physique doesn't happen overnight. Take regular measurements and photos. Keep a training diary. Because you see yourself every day, it's hard to notice the changes taking place in your body; having objective data provides perspective and allows you to impartially assess your progress.

Most important, don't be afraid to lift hard and heavy. The biggest reason women fail to change their shape is that they fail to sufficiently challenge their muscles. This is most often based on the misguided fear that heavy lifting will make them bulky. Trust me, this isn't the case.

Heavy loads are necessary to put sufficient strain on the muscles, which is a prerequisite for achieving a sculpted physique. Sure, you'll put on muscle, but it will be well distributed in all the right places. Your clothes will fit better. I've been lifting as heavy as I can possibly lift for the past 15 years, and I'm a size 4!

So put away the scale and let the mirror be your gauge. The reading on the scale is nothing more than a meaningless number. At the end of the day, it's not about how much you weigh but rather how you feel and how you look.

The most crucial ingredient for fitness success is a sound training program.

Brad Schoenfeld has solved that part of the equation in *Strong and Sculpted*. No one knows more about optimizing body composition than Brad. Here he provides a blueprint for getting into your best shape ever. His approach is scientifically based and draws on years of experience working with women of all shapes and sizes. Everything you need is laid out in an easy-to-follow manner. Whether your goal is to compete in a physique competition or simply to make the most of your genetic potential, this book will help you get there.

Yours in fitness,

Erin Stern
Two-time Figure Olympia champion

Acknowledgments

To my parents for instilling in me the importance of the scientific method from an early age and always encouraging me to pursue my dreams. I love you both eternally. Rest in peace.

To Bret Contreras and Alan Aragon for your help in reviewing the manuscript. You are true professionals who share a common passion for evidence-based practice and the pursuit of knowledge. I'm honored to call you the best of friends.

To Jessica Dillon for enriching my life and inspiring me to be better every day.

To my literary agent, Laura Blake Peterson, for your tireless efforts in making this project a reality. You are the best at what you do!

To the staff at Human Kinetics for believing in this project and putting in the resources to make it a success. In particular, I'd like to thank Michelle Maloney and Amy Stahl for facilitating the acquisition and providing insight on making the book the best it can be. Also a big thanks to Neil Bernstein for another terrific photo shoot.

Sculpting Your Ultimate Body

It started with a vision . . .

The year was 1998. At the time I was training a diverse array of women at my private fitness facility in Scarsdale, New York. My clients included several high-level physique athletes who competed in figure competitions. My sole focus was to get these women into peak condition; their competitive careers depended on it.

I approached the task like a rogue scientist: My training facility served as the research lab; my clients, the subjects. I experimented with a plethora of exercise routines; manipulated training variables in every way possible; found what worked, discarded what did not.

This trial-and-error process evolved into a system of training that proved highly successful, ultimately producing top-place finishes for many of my clients. Best of all, the system was designed as a template that could be customized to the needs and abilities of any woman interested in improving her physique—not just those with competitive aspirations.

Word about my training practices quickly got around. I developed a reputation as the go-to trainer for getting women of all shapes and sizes into their best possible condition. Magazines contacted me for quotes. I appeared as a regular guest on network TV shows. My waiting list for new clients soon exceeded six months.

Suddenly the vision came to me: My training system was ideally suited for a book. It was uncomplicated, easy to individualize, and applicable to the masses. Through the written word, I could show any woman willing to put in the effort how to look great without ever stepping foot in my fitness facility. In this way I could expand my reach across the country—across the world!

In November of 1999, the book, ultimately titled *Sculpting Her Body Perfect*, became a reality.

Almost immediately thereafter, it became a hit.

Magazines such as *Shape, Oxygen, Fitness*, and *Self* published excerpts and featured routines from the book in cover stories. I made appearances on numerous national U.S. television and radio programs. Book club rights were purchased; foreign rights were sold in multiple countries. A second edition of the book was published in 2002; a third edition followed in 2007. All told, combined domestic sales of all three editions well exceeded 100,000 copies, with thousands more sold internationally.

In the interim, I followed my passion to pursue higher education. I went on to earn a master's degree in kinesiology from the University of Texas and then a PhD with a focus on applied exercise science from Rocky Mountain University in

Utah. While continuing to consult with a select clientele on training and nutrition, I joined the world of academia as a professor in exercise science. I now head a lab that carries out controlled studies on strategies for optimizing body composition. To date, my research has produced over 80 published scientific papers that have appeared in many of the leading peer-reviewed exercise journals.

In conjunction with this metamorphosis from trainer to researcher, my training philosophy has been drastically altered. I came to realize that just because something works doesn't mean that something else might not work even better. Based on emerging research, I was compelled to reexamine the best practices for exercise program design. The upshot was a complete overhaul of the training system I once espoused, bringing practical application into line with modern science.

You hold in your hands the result of these efforts.

ABOUT THE STRONG AND SCULPTED PROGRAM

The Strong and Sculpted fitness plan is for women who are serious about getting into peak condition. It harnesses the latest scientific evidence along with years of time-tested practical experience to help you sculpt the body you've always desired. There are no gimmicky exercises, no unsubstantiated quick-fix solutions. Just tried-and-true training principles combined into a comprehensive program guaranteed to produce head-turning results.

The scientific basis of the program is supported with references, often from the research conducted in my lab. I encourage you to pull up the referenced studies and read through them at length. You'll gain a greater appreciation for the whys of the program. That said, this is a training manual, not a textbook. I therefore have opted to write in a conversational style that presents scientific concepts in a reader-friendly manner; jargon is kept to a minimum. Where applicable, sidebars shed light on relevant topics.

The program is integrated in stages based on training experience. The break-in phase is essentially a beginner routine (see chapter 7); the basic training phase is an intermediate-level routine (see chapter 8); and the advanced body-sculpting phase is for those who've spent a good amount of time lifting seriously (see chapter 9). The peak physique phase (see chapter 10) is intended to be selectively integrated into the advanced body-sculpting phase to achieve peak conditioning. A concept called periodization is employed to balance training and recovery, to help you optimize results while preventing the dreaded plateau.

As opposed to other popular fitness plans, the Strong and Sculpted program takes a total-body approach to training. All too often, women gravitate to inner- and outer-thigh machines and ab devices at the exclusion of exercises for other important major muscle groups. This is usually done with the misguided hope of spot-reducing body fat (see the sidebar Spot Reduction). Suffice to say, it's an ill-advised approach that will only lead you down the path to frustration. With the Strong and Sculpted program, you'll systematically develop a base of muscle and attain neuromuscular control. Once you've developed this foundation, you'll learn to employ more advanced body-sculpting techniques that ultimately allow you to focus on weak areas and achieve optimal shape and symmetry among your muscles.

A unique feature of this book is the categorization of exercises based on biomechanics and applied anatomical principles. These groupings allow you to

Spot Reduction

I get scores of e-mails each month asking some sort of variation of this question: What exercise can I do to reduce the fat in my [fill in the blank with a problem area]? No matter how the question is phrased, my answer is always the same: Sorry, but there is no such exercise.

Here's the reality: You can't spot-reduce fat. It's a physiological impossibility. All the sit-ups in the world won't give you a flat midsection; no amount of side leg lifts will preferentially slim down your saddle bags. In reality, trying to zap away your problem areas is literally an exercise in futility.

Here's why spot reduction doesn't work. When calories are consumed in abundance, your body converts the excess nutrients into fat-based compounds called triglycerides, which are then stored in cells called adipocytes (a.k.a. fat cells) that reside underneath the skin. Adipocytes are pliable storehouses that either shrink or expand to accommodate fatty deposits. They are present in virtually every part of the body including your face, your neck, and the soles of your feet.

When you exercise, triglycerides in adipocytes are broken back down into fatty acids, which are then transported via the blood to be used in target tissues for energy. Because fatty acids must travel through the circulatory system—a time-consuming event—it is just as efficient for your body to use fat from one area as it is another. (*Side note:* Muscles do contain their own internal fat stores called intramuscular triglycerides that can be used directly by the muscle for fuel, but these stores have no meaningful impact on your appearance.) Bottom line: The proximity of adipocytes to the working muscles is completely irrelevant from an energy standpoint.

---

easily piece together routines so that your exercises mesh properly. This foolproof system ensures that your muscles receive maximal stimulation with minimal overlap.

One thing's for certain: You'll train hard—probably harder than you've ever trained before. Embrace it! Whether you're lifting heavy, moderate, or light weights (and yes, you'll train through the spectrum of loading zones), a high degree of effort is key to maximizing your genetic potential.

HOW TO USE THIS PROGRAM

An old Chinese proverb says, "Give a man a fish, you feed him for a day; teach a man to fish, and you feed him for life." This sums up the approach I take with fitness. Exercise programming is specific to the person. Although the basic principles remain constant, women vary widely in their responses to training protocols. Pardon the pun, but a cookie-cutter routine therefore doesn't cut it. Any good training program can serve only as a template; it must then be customized based on individual response.

Accordingly, the goal of this book is to educate you on the hows and whys of program design so that you can tailor the routines to your needs and abilities. You should avoid the temptation to skip ahead to the training chapters. First read through the entire book cover to cover. Soak up the knowledge contained herein. Understand how the many variables affect muscle development. Appreciate how the routines are structured to bring about specific adaptations. The entire process won't take you more than a few hours; it will be time well spent.

From a training standpoint, start with the phase that corresponds to your current level of experience. Be honest with yourself on this front. Many women believe that they're advanced trainees because they've dabbled with lifting over the years. But time alone does not determine advanced status. More important is how serious and dedicated you are to training. I've known women who've lifted for six months and who are light-years ahead of others who've trained for a decade. When in doubt, start with the more rudimentary phase and progress only when you feel ready.

Also note that the sample routines merely provide suggestions for how to organize your routine. This is also true of the exercises. If a certain movement doesn't feel right to you or if you don't have access to a particular piece of equipment, simply substitute another exercise. Just make sure that the replacement is from the same category as the one listed. For example, say a particular routine calls for a barbell back squat but you don't have access to an Olympic bar. No problem. Simply perform a goblet squat instead. Although the two exercises aren't identical, they essentially work the same muscles in similar ways.

WHAT ABOUT BEING FUNCTIONAL?

A popular battle cry in some fitness circles is, *Train movements, not muscles*. The philosophy is based on the premise that muscles are designed to work in a coordinated fashion to produce functional movements. In theory, training with movement patterns similar to those involved in everyday activities promotes a functional body that is adept at facing life's physical challenges.

The flip side of this theory is that body-sculpting routines produce a nonfunctional body. Machine training, in particular, is vilified as functionally useless. Some even claim that by isolating muscles, you actually interfere with the coordination between them and thus impair functional capacity. On the surface, the rationale sounds logical. In actuality, it's baseless.

First and foremost, the ability to carry out activities of daily living (by all accounts the true determination of a functional body) is enhanced by increasing strength and power. If you get stronger and more powerful, your functional capacity will improve

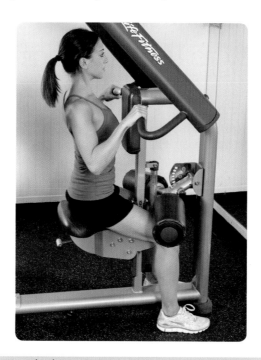

Machines can bring about functional adaptations.

regardless of how these attributes are attained. Want proof? In a classic research study, nine nursing home patients (average age 90 years!) performed three sets of leg extension exercises three times a week (Fiatarone et al., 1990). Now, you'd be hard-pressed to find an exercise that would appear to have less relevance to everyday movement patterns than the single-joint leg extension. The results? After eight weeks on the routine, leg strength in these subjects increased by 174 percent, and functional capacity correspondingly increased by 48 percent. Most impressive, two of the nine subjects were able to walk without the assistance of their canes! Think about it. Is anything more functional than being able to get around independently?

The belief that body-sculpting routines are nonfunctional is inherently flawed. Any well-structured program invariably includes numerous free weight and cable exercises that are carried out in three-dimensional space. Squats, presses, and rows are fundamental movements included in just about all functional routines—they're also body-sculpting staples. The contention that adding machine-based exercises to the mix somehow negatively affects functional capacity is not only unsupported by research, but also illogical from any scientific perspective.

From a practical standpoint, functional transfer takes place on a continuum, increasing as you move from machine-based exercises to free weight movements. But how this plays out in the everyday lives of women is another story. Certainly, an athlete would benefit from training specific to her sport. Even small improvements in on-the-field performance can be the difference between winning and losing a competition. For the average woman, however, these enhancements won't make a bit of difference in lifestyle. Have you ever seen a figure competitor who can't pick up her child? Or carry her groceries? Or rearrange furniture around her home? I didn't think so.

Bottom line: You'll not only look great after performing the Strong and Sculpted routine, but also be stronger and more powerful and, as a result, more functional.

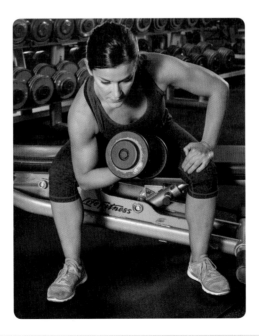

Free-weight exercises add to the functionality of the Strong and Sculpted routine.

WHAT CAN YOU EXPECT TO ACHIEVE?

Genes are what you inherit from your parents. They determine characteristics such as eye color, hair texture, and skin tone. From a physique standpoint, they determine your bone structure, muscle fiber typing, satellite cell activity, and many other factors that have direct relevance to your physical appearance. Approximately 25 to 50 percent of your body shape is genetically preordained.

To a certain extent, genetics are self-limiting. Short of radical surgery, you can't change your God-given DNA. What you were bestowed at birth is what you are stuck with throughout life. So if you are tall and large-framed, you're simply not going to fit into a size 2 dress no matter how much you diet and exercise. Nor will you get long and lean from performing a specific training regimen if you have short muscle bellies (see the sidebar Longer and Leaner?). But that's no reason to be discouraged.

The fact that only 25 to 50 percent of your body shape is genetically dictated means that you have the ability to alter appearance by anywhere from 50 to 75 percent! By using the body-sculpting principles and strategies outlined in this book, you can change your shape. I've worked with a number of high-level physique competitors who have come to me with what could only be described as average genetics. But through scientific training practices combined with hard work and dedication, these women overcame genetic deficiencies and placed in the top tiers of their competitive classes. If they can do it, so can you.

Now, it's true that people respond differently to training. I therefore can't tell you how much muscle you'll gain or what your body will look like following training. To a certain extent, this will depend on how you decide to sculpt your physique. What I can say with complete confidence is that if you put in the requisite effort, the program will help you achieve the upper limits of your genetic potential.

Excited to get started? Great! Put on your gym clothes, lace up your sneakers, and read on!

Longer and Leaner?

If you listen to the hype being dished out by certain fitness pros, you might be inclined to believe that exercising in a certain fashion can make you long and lean. The claim is most often attributed to a system of training called Pilates. Here's the rationale: Lifting weights is bad because it bulks up your muscles, making you tight and stiff. Pilates, on the other hand, supposedly lengthens muscles, giving you a dancer's physique that is willowy and flowing.

Pretty amazing, huh? Think about it. Increasing the length of your muscles would not only make you leaner, but also taller and more statuesque. Heck, sign me up now!

One little problem . . . the prospect of becoming longer and leaner is a physiological impossibility.

It can't happen. The fact is, your genetic structure is inherent. Every muscle in your body has a predetermined structure predicated on such factors as fiber type composition, tendon insertions, and muscle belly length. You simply cannot alter these properties unless you somehow find a mad scientist who's invented a new form of gene therapy. Sorry, but that's reality.

Now, this isn't to say that Pilates or similar disciplines don't have a place in a workout routine. If integrated into a regimented exercise program, such training can enhance fitness components. But don't fall prey to marketing propaganda: Whether or not you're long and lean depends on your genes, not your training regimen.

2

The Strong and Sculpted Program

You've no doubt heard this adage: "Those who fail to plan, plan to fail." With respect to fitness, truer words were never spoken. The probability that you'll achieve your physique-related goals without a solid blueprint for success is slim to none.

Yet all too often, people go to the gym with no sense of a game plan. Some adhere to the same old routine day in and day out without regard for progression. Others wander around aimlessly deciding what to do next. The result for all these lifters is a failure to attain their desired results.

Planning an exercise program is best accomplished by using a technique called periodization. Periodization refers to the planned manipulation of program variables to optimize a given fitness outcome. Simply stated, it's a strategy to keep progressing in your fitness efforts without hitting a plateau.

The genesis of periodization can be traced back to the 1950s when Russian scientists devised the concept to prepare athletes for Olympic events. Training was segmented into distinct cycles that corresponded to given fitness components. The cycle traditionally began with a hypertrophy or endurance phase, progressed to a strength phase, and then culminated in a power phase. The Russian model, popularly known as linear periodization, was designed to take place over a four-year period—the time between Olympic competitions. When properly implemented, the athlete would peak just in time for the contest. Perhaps it should come as no surprise that the Soviet Union dominated in terms of the number of Olympic medals won in the years following the implementation of periodized training.

Although linear periodization proved to be highly successful, strength coaches from around the world began experimenting with alternative forms of the model. The concept of undulating periodization was soon born. Rather than use progressive cycles focusing on different fitness components, the undulating model varies training variables within short time frames. Most often, this involves rotating heavy, moderate, and light training days, generally over the course of a week or two.

Despite much debate, there is no best method for periodization; all of the models can produce excellent results. The common thread is that all of the models involve the manipulation of training program variables, including volume, frequency, loading, exercise selection, intensity of effort, and rest intervals. As long as proper progression and adequate recovery is built in to the scheme, many approaches are viable depending on your ultimate goal.

The Strong and Sculpted program, a hybrid of linear and undulating periodization models, has proven highly successful for getting women into top shape. A modified daily undulating periodization model is used for the basic training and advanced body-sculpting phases (chapters 8 and 9, respectively), whereas the peak physique routine is essentially a modified linear cycle (chapter 10).

If this sounds intimidating, don't worry; I keep things simple here. There are no complicated formulas, no convoluted training schemes. It's all laid out in an easy-to-follow fashion. To provide context for the program, the following are overviews of the training variables and how they are manipulated to optimize results.

VOLUME

Volume of training pertains to the amount of work completed over a given training period (usually on a per-session or per-week basis). Volume can be expressed in a couple of ways. Commonly, it is specific to repetitions. Thus, multiplying the number of reps by the number of sets performed over the time period in question provides a measure of training volume. Perhaps a more relevant gauge of volume can be obtained by factoring in the amount of weight you lifted as well. In this scenario you multiply reps × sets × load. The product, called volume-load, gives a true sense of the total work accomplished during training.

Although volume is widely regarded as playing an essential role in muscle development, some fitness pros claim otherwise. They subscribe to a theory called high-intensity training (HIT), which proposes that performing a single set of an exercise to failure is all that's required to maximize muscular adaptations. According to HIT theory, performing additional sets is not only superfluous, but actually counterproductive to results.

So who's right?

Without question, single-set training is an effective strategy to build muscle. For those with limited time to devote to working out, it's a viable option. That

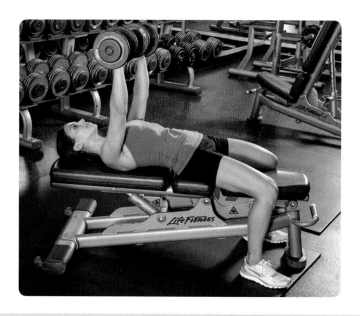

Proper manipulation of program variables is essential to maximizing results.

said, if your goal is to maximize muscle development, HIT simply doesn't do the trick. You need a higher training volume.

Substantially higher.

Research shows a clear dose–response relationship between training volume and muscle growth. Simply stated, this means that as the volume of training increases, so does hypertrophy—at least up to a point. A meta-analysis by Krieger (2010) published in the *Journal of Strength and Conditioning Research* demonstrated just how important volume is to muscular adaptation. Data from all pertinent studies were pooled for analysis, and a specialized statistical technique called regression was employed to rule out confounding issues. The findings? Effect size (a measure of the meaningfulness of results) was over 40 percent greater when multiple sets were performed compared to single sets.

Bottom line: If your goal is to maximize your genetic potential, higher volumes are a must.

Now, before you start thinking that having a great body requires that you spend all your waking hours in the gym, understand that the dose–response relationship follows an inverted-U curve (see figure 2.1). This implies that increases in volume result in greater gains up to a certain threshold. Once the threshold is reached, further increases in volume have diminishing returns; when taken to excess, volume increases ultimately lead to an overtrained state (see the sidebar Understanding Overtraining, which addresses the detriments of exercising too much). The goal, therefore, is to perform just enough volume to max out your gains.

Easy, right? Not quite.

Unfortunately, there is no one-size-fits-all prescription for training volume. To an extent it depends on the person. Genetics enters into the equation. So do lifestyle factors such as nutritional status, training experience, stress levels, and sleep patterns. A fair amount of experimentation is required to determine your particular optimal volume levels.

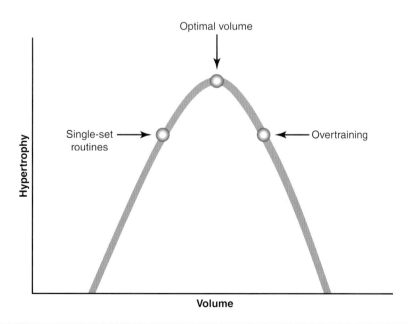

Figure 2.1 Dose–response relationship between volume and hypertrophy.

That said, there is a benefit to manipulating volume over time. Ideally, this is accomplished by instituting periodic high-volume training phases to promote functional overreaching. These overreaching phases should be relatively brief and involve pushing your body to its limits and then pulling back in volume and intensity so that you don't become overtrained. When properly implemented, the strategy promotes a supercompensated response that optimizes muscle development.

Intense training also requires that you incorporate regular deload periods (generally lasting a week) into your program. Deloads facilitate the recuperation and restoration of bodily systems by reducing training volume (along with intensity). In this way, you come back strong and refreshed, and progress continues on an upward trend. The frequency of deloads again depends on your particular response to training. A good rule of thumb is to deload once a month or so, and then adjust the frequency accordingly.

Although the total volume of a program is an important metric, you also need to consider the volume per muscle group. Larger muscles require more volume to fully stimulate all fibers. The lats, traps, pectorals, glutes, and quads fall into this category. Moreover, certain smaller muscles such as the biceps and triceps are worked extensively during multijoint pushing and pulling movements (e.g., presses and rows). Hence, these muscles don't need as much direct work to maximize development.

The Strong and Sculpted program manages volume throughout each phase, both overall and with respect to individual muscle groups. The program takes into account your training level, progressively increasing volume as you gain experience with lifting. Once you get to advanced status, the peak physique phase takes your physique to its ultimate potential.

Understanding Overtraining

Overtraining is a fairly common exercise-related affliction. It has been estimated that overtraining affects as much as 10 percent of all people who exercise on a regular basis. Because of a lack of understanding of the condition, it often ends up going undiagnosed.

Simply stated, overtraining results from performing too much strenuous physical activity. However, the exact threshold for overtraining varies from person to person. People respond differently to exercise. Some can tolerate large volumes of training; whereas others, much less. What's more, factors such as nutritional status, sleeping patterns, hormonal concentrations, and previous training experience all affect recuperative capacity and, therefore, the point at which overtraining rears its ugly head.

Overtraining can be classified into two categories: localized and systemic. Although both have the same origin (too much intense exercise), their repercussions are quite different. Of the two subtypes, localized overtraining is by far the most common. As the name implies, it is localized to a specific muscle or muscle group without affecting other bodily systems. It generally strikes those who are involved in serious strength training programs, especially bodybuilders, powerlifters, and fitness competitors.

Localized overtraining is bound to occur when the same muscle group is trained too frequently in a given time span. This can even happen using a split routine, in which different muscle groups are trained on different days. You see, during the performance of most exercises, synergistic interactions occur among muscle groups. The biceps, for instance, are integrally involved in the performance of back maneuvers; the shoulders and triceps are involved in many exercises for the chest, as are the glutes and hamstrings during compound leg movements. ⟶

Other muscles function as stabilizers: The abdominals and erector spinae (the muscles of the low back), in particular, help to provide stability in a variety of upper- and lower-body exercises, contracting statically throughout each move. The fact is, when a muscle is repeatedly subjected to intense physical stress (even on a secondary level) without being afforded adequate rest, the rate at which microtrauma occurs outpaces the reparation process. The result is impaired localized muscular strength and development.

Systemic overtraining, on the other hand, is more complex, and potentially more serious, than localized overtraining. As the name implies, it is all encompassing, acting on the body as a whole. Commonly referred to as overtraining syndrome (OTS, for short), it affects thousands of exercisers each year. Strength and endurance athletes are equally at risk.

In almost all cases, OTS causes the body to enter a catabolic state. Catabolism is mediated by an increased production of cortisol—a stress hormone secreted by the adrenal cortex—which exerts its influence at the cellular level, impeding muscular repair and function. Making matters worse, a corresponding decrease in testosterone production often occurs, depleting the body of its most potent anabolic stimulus. These factors combine to inhibit protein synthesis and accelerate muscle protein breakdown. Not only does this result in a cessation of muscular development, but it also makes the body less efficient at using fat for fuel—a double whammy that wreaks havoc on body composition.

In addition, because of a depletion of glutamine stores, OTS suppresses the body's immune system. Glutamine is the major source of energy for immune cells. A steady supply is necessary for their proper function. However, glutamine levels are rapidly exhausted when exercise volume is high. Without an adequate amount of fuel, the immune system loses its ability to produce antibodies such as lymphocytes, leukocytes, and cytokines. Ultimately, the body's capacity to fight viral and bacterial infections becomes impaired, leading to an increased incidence of infirmity.

Following are some of the symptoms of OTS. If you experience two or more of these symptoms, you very well might be systemically overtrained. If symptoms persist, get plenty of sleep and don't resume training until you feel mentally and physically ready.

- Increased resting heart rate
- Increased resting blood pressure
- Decreased exercise performance
- Decreased appetite
- Decreased desire to work out
- Increased incidence of injuries
- Increased incidence of infections and flu-like symptoms
- Increased irritability and depression

FREQUENCY

Frequency of training refers to the number of exercise sessions performed over a given period of time, usually a week. It is generally believed that at least three lifting sessions per week are necessary for optimizing body composition, but a greater frequency can enhance results, at least up to a point. That said, train too frequently for too long, and you'll end up overtrained.

The solution: periodize your training frequency so that you progressively increase it over a given period of time.

In addition to the number of total weekly training sessions, another frequency-related consideration is how much time to allow before working the same muscle group again. Make no mistake, training a muscle group too often is detrimental to results. As an analogy, say you got sunburned after spending time on a tropical beach. It wouldn't be prudent to go back to the beach the next morning, right? Doing so would only increase the severity of the burn. But allow a few days to pass and the burn will subside. Even better, your skin adapts by producing more melanin so that future exposure to the sun will result in a tan instead of a burn.

What does a suntan have to do with resistance training frequency? Intense lifting results in structural damage to the muscle fibers. During recovery, the body repairs this damage so that the muscle comes back bigger and stronger for the next bout. But if you hit the same muscle hard before the process has fully run its course, you deprive it of the opportunity to repair. In effect, muscle tissue is broken down at a greater rate than the body can rebuild it, ultimately compromising muscle development (i.e., localized overtraining).

A good rule of thumb is to allow a minimum of 48 hours between exercises for the same muscle group. This is the approximate amount of time that protein synthesis remains elevated following a resistance training bout. You also need to keep in mind the contribution of secondary muscle movers to exercise performance. Upper-body pushing exercises such as the bench press and shoulder press heavily involve the triceps, whereas pulling movements such as lat pulldowns and chin-ups require substantial contribution from the biceps. Routines should therefore be structured so that all muscles receiving extensive stimulation in a workout are afforded adequate recovery time to reduce the risk of localized overtraining.

Perhaps the most appropriate reason for altering training frequency is to regulate volume. Provided that volume remains constant within each training session, a greater workout frequency necessarily results in a greater weekly volume (e.g., six weekly workouts produce a higher volume than three workouts of the same composition). Accordingly, a greater frequency increases the potential for overtraining assuming that the per-session training volume is maintained. It's therefore imprudent to consistently train on successive days over long periods of time, even if individual muscles are afforded sufficient rest between workout sessions.

The Strong and Sculpted plan progressively increases frequency as you gain training experience. This allows your body to acclimate to the heightened stresses from more frequent training sessions. In the early phases, you'll use a total-body routine so that each muscle is trained multiple times per week. This enhances the neural response, facilitating your ability to hone your exercise technique. In the advanced phases, a split routine allows you to perform a greater volume while providing proper recovery between sessions. The peak physique phase is the ultimate in high-frequency training. It is intended to bring about functional overreaching in a manner that optimizes muscle development. But because the frequency (and thus volume) is so high, it's a brief phase lasting several weeks that should be performed only every few months.

LOADING

The amount of weight you lift—called the intensity of load—is an important consideration for building muscle. Intensity of load is generally expressed as a percentage of one-repetition maximum (1RM)—the amount of weight you can lift once but not a second time while maintaining proper form. For example, say your 1RM for the back squat is 100 pounds (45 kg). If you perform this lift at 75 percent of 1RM, you'd be lifting 75 pounds (34 kg). Alternatively, intensity of loading can be expressed by a given repetition range. For example, an 8RM would be a load you can lift eight times but not nine.

Now, it should be apparent from these definitions that the term *heavy* is specific to the intensity of load; the closer you get to a 1RM, the heavier the weight will be. However, the effort you put into a set will affect your perception of a weight's heaviness. For instance, if you perform a set of squats at your 20RM, the first few reps will be easy and thus feel light. By the time you reach your 10th rep, that same weight will be more challenging; and once you reach that 20th rep, the load will feel extremely heavy. Thus, *heavy* and *light* are relative terms that need to be understood in proper context. From our standpoint, we use these terms specifically as they relate to intensity of load; a heavy weight means that you are lifting close to your 1RM.

From a loading perspective, we can create various loading zones that correspond to repetition ranges: heavy (3-5RM), medium (8-12RM), and light (15+RM). This method of categorization provides a framework for program design because the loading zones involve the use of different energy systems and tax your neuromuscular system in different ways. Here's the lowdown on how each zone contributes to building muscle.

Heavy-load sessions in a low-rep range are necessary to maximize strength, primarily through improvements in neural efficiency (i.e., recruitment, rate coding, and synchronization). Stronger muscles allow you to use heavier weights—and thus generate greater muscular tension—in the medium-repetition range that is considered optimal for muscle building. If you can increase muscle tension without compromising the number of reps performed, you're setting the stage for enhanced muscle development. It also is believed that lifting heavy loads helps in the conditioning of stubborn high-threshold motor units (the ones associated

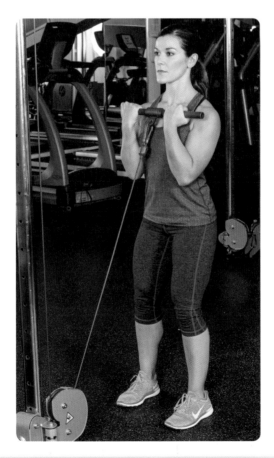

Training through a spectrum of rep ranges enhances muscle development.

with the largest Type II fibers), so that they are recruited at lower percentages of 1RM. The upshot is that you stimulate the full spectrum of Type II fibers during medium-rep training.

Medium-load training is a staple in body-sculpting routines. These loads are heavy enough to not only promote substantial mechanical tension, but also maintain the tension for a sufficient time to stimulate the full spectrum of available fibers in working muscles. In addition, the use of medium loads generates considerable metabolic stress. The associated buildup of metabolites influences growth in multiple ways, including the production of growth factors, increased cell swelling, and greater muscle fiber activation. Better yet, the combination of these factors is believed to have a synergistic effect on muscle development, increasing gains over and above what can be achieved from either of these mechanisms alone. Accordingly, medium-load training has come to be known as the hypertrophy rep range.

Finally, the use of lighter loads with high reps has several benefits from a body-sculpting standpoint. For one, it increases your lactate threshold—the point at which lactic acid rapidly begins to accumulate in working muscles. An excessive buildup of lactic acid inhibits muscle contraction, reducing the number of reps you can perform. Higher-rep training counteracts lactic acid accumulation by increasing the number of capillaries (tiny blood vessels that facilitate the exchange of nutrients and metabolic waste) and heightening muscle-buffering capacity, allowing you to perform an extra rep or two when pushing to failure. Moreover, the increase in capillaries enhances the delivery of substances (e.g., oxygen, hormones, amino acids) to bodily tissues, promoting better recovery following an intense workout.

In addition to these indirect effects, training in a high-rep range directly enhances muscle development by targeting your endurance-oriented Type I fibers. The greater time under load associated with high-rep training keeps Type I fibers activated to a greater extent than when training with low- to medium-rep ranges, providing the necessary stimulus for their growth. And despite the claims of some fitness pros, Type I fibers are important in overall muscle development (Ogborn & Schoenfeld, 2014).

Research from my lab indicates that combining loading zones over the course of a training program maximizes muscle development (Schoenfeld, Wilson, et al., 2014). The Strong and Sculpted program takes full advantage of this strategy. Loading zones are manipulated in a systematic fashion. You'll train through the full continuum of rep ranges during the majority of the program, while focusing on the hypertrophy range to achieve your peak physique. And if by chance you're worried about getting too bulky from lifting hard and heavy, see the sidebar Bulking Up.

EXERCISE SELECTION

Most lifters have a limited number of favorite exercises that are staples in their routines. That's human nature. However, although it's OK to have your old standbys, they shouldn't be performed at the exclusion of other movements. In fact, varying exercises through a multiplanar, multiangled approach is essential to fully develop complete symmetry both within and between muscles.

The importance of variety is apparent from basic functional anatomy (see figures 2.2 and 2.3 for full-body muscle illustrations). Muscles often have diverse

Bulking Up

I want to tone, not bulk!

As a fitness trainer, educator, and researcher, I hear women utter these words every day. The sad fact is that the majority of women fear gaining any appreciable amount of muscle. This mind-set is largely a product of the society we live in. From Madison Avenue to Hollywood, women have long been glamorized in the form of stick-thin waifs. Thigh gap and protruding ribs are seen as physical attributes.

Fortunately, times are beginning to change.

Resistance training is steadily gaining popularity among women. In increasing numbers, women are embracing the fact that a strong body is a feminine body. A new era has emerged in which sculpted muscle is becoming the new skinny. The fact that you're reading this book indicates that you're squarely in this camp.

Still, the concern of getting bulky from lifting continues to pervade the female psyche, even in women who lift weights. All too often, fitness professionals feed into the toning mentality by telling women to train only with light weights. One popular celebrity trainer has gone as far as to say that women who lift anything heavier than 2 pounds (about 1 kg) risk developing bulging muscles.

Hogwash!

Pure and simple, the aversion to lifting heavy weights is based on beliefs that are completely unfounded. Although the amount of weight lifted is directly related to strength gains, going heavier doesn't necessarily build more muscle. Recent work from my lab shows that similar muscle growth can be achieved using even very light loads provided that they are lifted with a high degree of effort (Schoenfeld, Peterson, et al., 2015). Ultimately, muscle growth comes down to challenging your muscles; the amount of load is somewhat secondary to the process.

As far as bulking up, that should be the least of your worries. The vast majority of women don't have the ability to pack on slabs of muscle. This is largely a function of hormones. Levels of circulating testosterone, the primary muscle-building hormone, are tenfold greater in men than in women. If anything, you'll have to work your tail off to achieve what is commonly considered a sculpted look with such low testosterone production.

What about the female bodybuilders you see in the magazines? They are anomalies. For one, they have extraordinary genetics suited to building muscle. We're talking the top 1/100th of 1 percent of the population. What's more, they invariably are chemically enhanced; no matter how great your genetics is, you can't win a pro bodybuilding show without taking performance-enhancing drugs. All things considered, you have a better chance of seeing Bigfoot drinking a beer in Central Park than looking like one of these competitors from lifting weights.

Bottom line: There is no reason to fear heavy training. In fact, it's an important component to achieve the body you've always desired. It's not going to bulk you up, at least in the context of the program in this book. So ditch the pink dumbbell mentality and, regardless of the amount of weight used, train with a high level of effort.

Now admittedly, *bulky* is a subjective term. Some women might believe that they are overly muscular when others perceive them as slim and shapely. How you choose to look is a personal decision; no one should impose an ideal of aesthetics on you. The good news is that it's much easier to lose muscle than it is to gain it. So if at any point you start to feel that a certain area of your body is getting too muscular, simply cut back on training that muscle group. In short order the size of that muscle will decrease and, like a true physique artist, you'll ultimately sculpt the body that you desire.

attachments to optimize leverage for varying movement patterns. For example, the deltoids are subdivided into three distinct heads that carry out separate functions: the anterior head flexes the shoulder (raises the arm forward); the middle head abducts the shoulder (raises the arm to the side); and the posterior head horizontally extends the shoulder (moves the arm away from the midline of the body from a position where it's parallel to the floor). These unique functions can be trained by performing a front raise, lateral raise, and bent fly. In this way, you target each respective deltoid head so that all fibers are maximally stimulated.

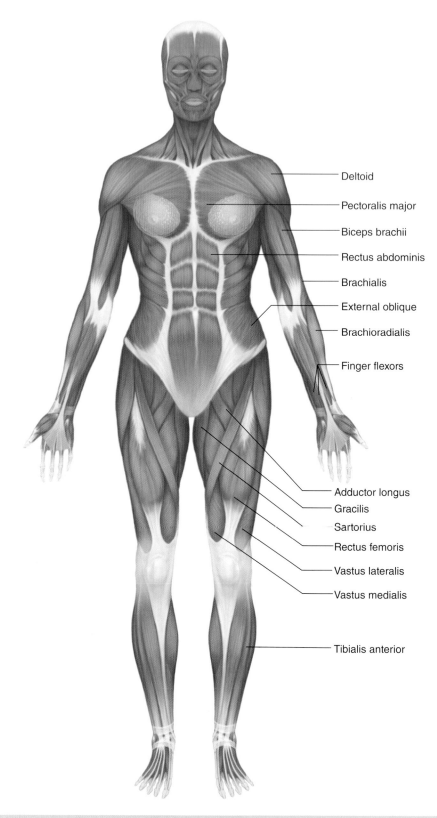

Deltoid

Pectoralis major

Biceps brachii

Rectus abdominis

Brachialis

External oblique

Brachioradialis

Finger flexors

Adductor longus

Gracilis

Sartorius

Rectus femoris

Vastus lateralis

Vastus medialis

Tibialis anterior

Figure 2.2 Full-body female anatomy (anterior view).

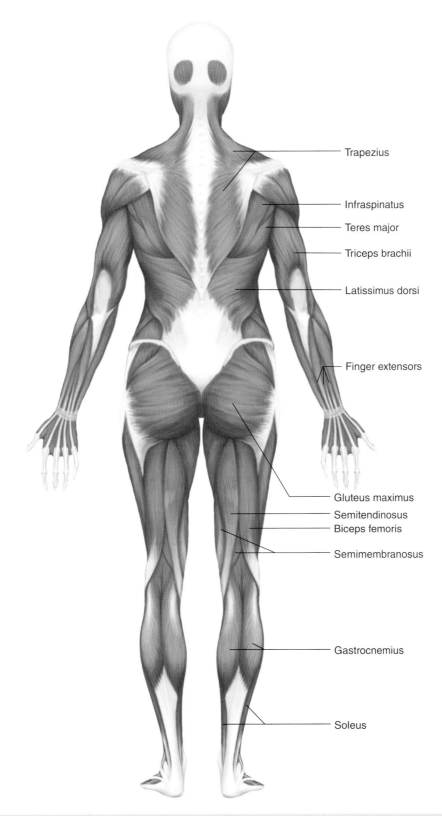

Trapezius

Infraspinatus

Teres major

Triceps brachii

Latissimus dorsi

Finger extensors

Gluteus maximus

Semitendinosus

Biceps femoris

Semimembranosus

Gastrocnemius

Soleus

Figure 2.3 Full-body female anatomy (posterior view).

OK, so perhaps this isn't news to you. What you might not know, however, is that it's actually possible to target portions of the same muscle fiber! Contrary to what was once thought, fibers don't necessarily span the entire length of the muscle from origin to insertion. Rather, they are often segmented into neuro-muscular compartments, each of which is activated by its own nerve branch. In fact, a majority of the large muscles in the body are compartmentalized in this fashion. This has wide-ranging implications for body sculpting. For example, a recent study from my lab found that the leg curl (a knee-dominant exercise) activated the lower aspect of the hamstrings to a much greater extent than the stiff-leg deadlift (a hip-dominant exercise) (Schoenfeld, Contreras, et al., 2015). The findings suggest that the partitioning of muscles provides a mechanism for their greater regional-specific activation.

Importantly, an emerging body of research indicates that the selective acti-vation of different areas of a muscle is consistent with where growth occurs in that muscle (Wakahara et al., 2012, 2013). Translation: Activating aspects of a given muscle can influence the extent of its development. A key takeaway here is that optimal body-sculpting results can be achieved only by working all aspects of all the major muscles, and this can be achieved only by performing a variety of exercises.

With respect to exercise selection, the concept of variety needs to be expanded beyond simply performing an array of exercises; you also need to take into account how these movements interact with each other. Basic kinesiology dictates that certain exercises are complementary, working synergistically to produce optimal results. Factors such as the angle of pull, plane of movement, length–ten-sion relationship, and number of joints involved influence how effectively you work a given muscle. Unfortunately, most lifters do not fully comprehend these complexities and continue to haphazardly string together a series of exercises without regard to how they mesh.

The good news is that you don't have to be an exercise physiologist to create a cohesive routine; the Strong and Sculpted plan takes all the guesswork out of exercise selection. You won't have to worry about deciding which movements mesh best; I've done all the legwork for you. Exercises for each muscle group are categorized based on applied kinesiological principles. Simply choose from the categories as directed, and you're guaranteed to effectively target the areas of the muscle complex you are working on that day. The result will be complete development of your physique over the course of the training program.

INTENSITY OF EFFORT

Of all the exercise variables, none is more important than intensity of effort (i.e., how hard you work out). With respect to resistance training, effort is dictated by the overload principle. Simply stated, this means that your muscles must be challenged beyond their physical capacity in order to develop.

By nature, the human body doesn't like change. It strives to maintain stabil-ity—a phenomenon called homeostasis. Nudging your body from its homeostatic state requires progressively higher levels of effort; otherwise, it is not sufficiently challenged and thus has no impetus to adapt. From a muscle-building standpoint, this implies that if you don't consistently push your body beyond its comfort zone, you'll fall short of achieving your genetic potential.

A lack of effort is the biggest downfall I see in women's quest for better bodies; they simply don't train hard enough to effect change in their physiques. Many seem to believe that using light weights is the best way to "tone up," and thus they never provide enough of an impetus for their muscles to develop. (I've actually seen trainees talking on cell phones and reading magazines while doing exercises such as leg presses and biceps curls!) Needless to say, such an approach is destined to lead to substandard results.

On the other hand, pushing yourself too hard too often is equally as misguided. Research shows that such an approach ultimately impairs anabolic hormonal levels while chronically elevating the stress hormone cortisol-factors associated with over-training and psychological burnout (Fry & Kraemer, 1997; Izquierdo et al., 2006). The upshot is that progress slows to a crawl or, worse, regresses to the point that you actually lose precious muscle. I liken this phenomenon to consistently flooring the gas pedal in your car; if the RPMs stay in the red zone for a prolonged period, eventually the engine is going to conk out. Well, your body is no different. It can handle high intensities of effort for limited periods of time. But push the envelope beyond a certain point, and you end up overtrained.

The Strong and Sculpted plan periodizes intensity of effort so that it is systematically varied over time. At least some of your sets will be taken to the point of momentary muscular failure—the point at which you are physically unable to perform another rep. If you are not used to this approach, you'll have to alter your mind-set to ensure that you attain true failure. It is human nature to seek pleasure and avoid pain. Pushing your body beyond the pain threshold is uncomfortable and thus undesirable for most. Make sure that your mind isn't giving up before your body does. To achieve optimal results, you must disregard the pain threshold and completely fatigue your target muscles.

To gauge intensity of effort, you'll use the reps-to-failure (RTF) scale, originally proposed by Hackett et al. (2012), which is summarized in table 2.1. As the name implies, effort is based on the number of reps you perceive you are from the point of muscular failure. I like the scale for its simplicity. The ratings range from 0 to 4, in which 4 indicates that you stop four reps short of failure, 3 indicates that you stop three reps short of failure, and so on. A rating of 0 indicates that you go all out and thus are unable to perform another repetition.

REST INTERVALS

The amount of time taken between sets (a.k.a. rest intervals) is an often-overlooked training variable. Most lifters give it very little regard. Standard practice is to perform a set and then meander around the gym and chat it up with no regard for time.

Table 2.1   Reps-to-Failure Scale

RTF	Description
0	Muscle failure: cannot perform another concentric rep with proper form
1	Set is stopped 1 rep short of failure
2	Set is stopped 2 reps short of failure
3	Set is stopped 3 reps short of failure
4	Set is stopped 4 reps short of failure

The question is, Are there any benefits to periodizing the time spent between sets?

To date, only a few research studies have investigated the effects of manipulating rest intervals on muscle development. Based on the limited research, the length of rest between sets doesn't appear to make much, if any, difference in this regard. It would therefore seem that you can select a rest period that allows you to exert the needed effort into your next set without compromising results.

Well, not so fast . . .

Rest intervals can be classified into three broad categories: short (30 seconds or less), moderate (1 to 2 minutes), and long (3 minutes or more). Short rest intervals enhance metabolic stress. If you limit your time between sets, metabolite accumulation skyrockets. Not only does this enhance your body's anabolic environment, but it also makes your muscles more impervious to lactic acid—factors beneficial for both muscular endurance and size. The downside is that the time is insufficient to regain your strength, which compromises mechanical tension and thus muscle-building capacity. The best use of short rest intervals is therefore in high-rep work, in which the performance-oriented goal is to enhance local muscle endurance and raise your lactate threshold.

Alternatively, longer rest intervals are beneficial for strength gains because they facilitate complete muscular recovery after performing a set. This allows you to train with your heaviest weight within a given repetition range, ensuring that the tension in your muscles remains high during the ensuing set. However, metabolic stress dissipates as the length of a rest interval increases, reducing its effects on muscle building. Hence, long rest intervals are best employed during low-rep work in which strength is the primary desired outcome. The associated strength increases can translate into an enhanced ability to use heavier loads during moderate-rep training, which in turn spurs muscle growth.

Moderate rest intervals provide a compromise between short and long ones. You regain a majority of your strength after about two minutes rest—enough to maintain high levels of muscular tension. Better yet, regimented training with moderate rest periods evokes adaptations that allow you to sustain performance with even higher percentages of your 1RM—up to 90 percent of maximal strength capacity! Moderate rest intervals also are associated with substantial metabolic stress because training is recommended before the accumulated metabolites can be fully removed. Although it may seem that moderate rest intervals provide the best of both worlds, neither mechanical tension nor metabolic stress is optimized. Thus, the approach is best used during moderate-rep work, in which the focus is directly on muscle development; a combination of high mechanical tension and elevated metabolic stress is believed to provide a synergistic effect on this outcome.

GOING FORWARD

Now that you have an understanding of how to manipulate variables, it's time to put the concepts together into a cohesive training program. The next three chapters provide descriptions of exercises for all the major muscles that can be incorporated into your routines. Go through these chapters with a particular focus on how the exercises fit into the categories for each muscle group. You'll then have the proper context for implementing them in the phases of the Strong and Sculpted program found in chapters 7 through 10.

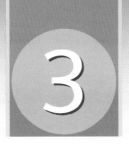

Exercises for the Shoulders and Arms

This chapter describes and illustrates exercises for the muscles of the shoulders and arms. Read the descriptions carefully, and scrutinize the photos to ensure proper form. I have provided expert tips for each of these movements to optimize your training performance. Remember that exercises are merely tools, or a means to an end—in this case, for enhancing muscular development. If an exercise does not feel right to you, simply substitute it for a comparable move.

SHOULDER EXERCISES

Exercises for the shoulders are divided into the following three categories (see table 3.1):

- Category 1 comprises multijoint overhead pressing exercises and upright rowing.
- Category 2 comprises single-joint frontal plane exercises for the shoulder musculature that target the middle head of the deltoid.
- Category 3 comprises single-joint transverse plane exercises for the shoulder musculature that target the posterior head of the deltoid.

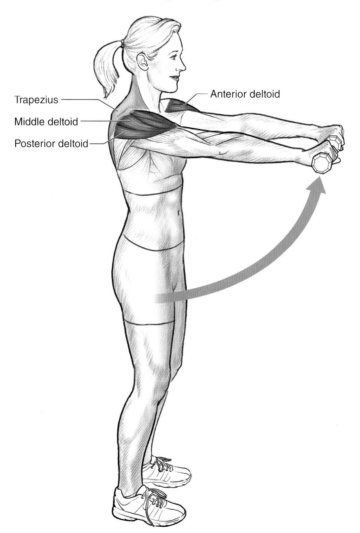

Table 3.1 Shoulder Exercises by Category

Category 1	Category 2	Category 3
Dumbbell shoulder press	Dumbbell lateral raise	Dumbbell seated bent reverse fly
Military press	Cable lateral raise	Cable reverse fly
Dumbbell upright row	Machine lateral raise	Cable kneeling bent reverse fly
Machine shoulder press		Machine rear deltoid fly
Cable upright row		

DUMBBELL SHOULDER PRESS

This move targets the deltoids, with an emphasis on the front delts. Secondary emphasis is on the upper trapezius and triceps.

Shoulder Category 1

START

Sit at the edge of a flat bench or chair. Grasp two dumbbells and bring the weights to shoulder level with your palms facing away from your body.

MOVEMENT

Press the dumbbells upward and in, allowing them to touch together directly over your head. Contract your deltoids and then return the dumbbells along the same arc to the start position.

EXPERT TIP

Don't arc the weights outward as you press; this increases stress to the connective tissue in the shoulder joint.

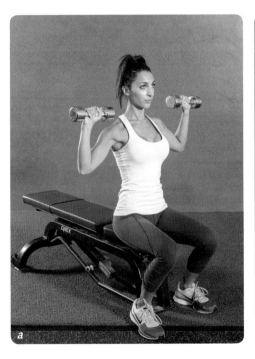
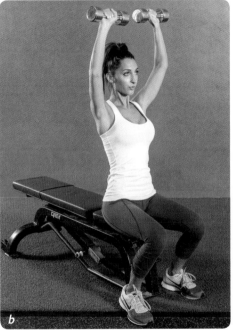

MILITARY PRESS

This move targets the shoulders, particularly the front delts. Secondary emphasis is on the upper trapezius and triceps.

Shoulder Category 1

START

Sit at the edge of a flat bench or chair. Grasp a barbell and bring it to the level of your upper chest with your palms facing away from your body.

MOVEMENT

Press the barbell directly upward and over your head, contracting your deltoids at the top of the move. Return the bar along the same path to the start position.

EXPERT TIPS

- The elbows should remain forward, not flared, throughout the move to maintain movement in the sagittal plane.
- If you don't have access to a power rack, you will need to lift (i.e., clean) the bar to shoulder level to begin the exercise.

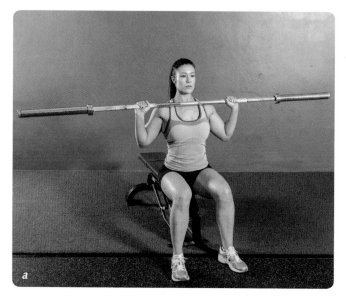
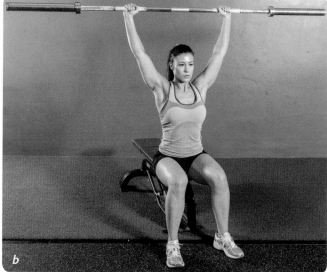

DUMBBELL UPRIGHT ROW

This move targets the middle delts with secondary emphasis on the biceps.

Shoulder Category 1

START

Grasp two dumbbells with a shoulder-width grip. Allow your arms to hang down from your shoulders with your palms facing in toward your body. Assume a comfortable stance and keep your knees slightly bent.

MOVEMENT

Keeping your elbows higher than your wrists at all times, raise the dumbbells upward along the line of your body until your upper arms approach shoulder level. Contract your delts and lower the weights along the same path back to the start position.

EXPERT TIPS

- Be careful not to lift your elbows beyond parallel to the floor. Doing so can lead to shoulder impingement, causing rotator cuff injury.
- Keep the weights as close to your body as possible throughout the movement.

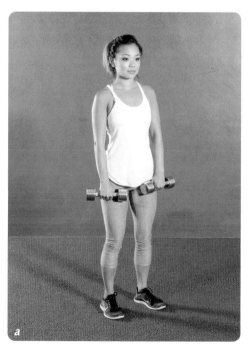 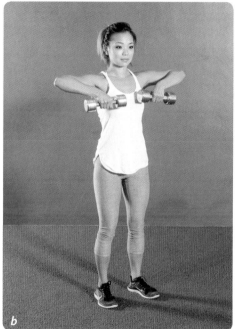

MACHINE SHOULDER PRESS

This move targets the deltoids, with an emphasis on the front delts. Secondary emphasis is on the upper trapezius and the triceps.

Shoulder Category 1

START

Sit upright in the seat of a shoulder press machine with your back supported by the pad. Grasp the handles of the machine with your palms facing away from your body and your elbows flared out to the sides. Adjust the seat height so that the handles are slightly above the level of your shoulders.

MOVEMENT

Keeping your elbows flared, press the handles directly up and over your head, contracting your deltoids at the top of the move. Return the handles to the start position.

EXPERT TIPS

- Don't lock your elbows at the top of the move; doing so reduces tension to the target muscles.
- Keep your elbows flared to the sides as you lift; allowing them to move forward changes the scope of the exercise.

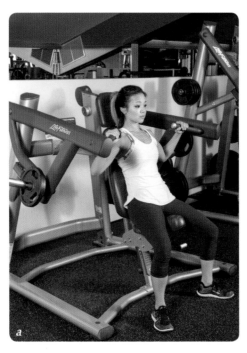
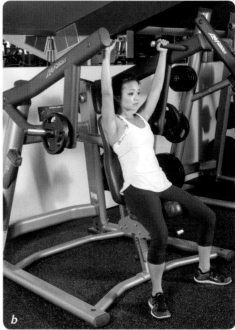

CABLE UPRIGHT ROW

This move targets the middle delts and places secondary emphasis on the biceps.

Shoulder Category 1

START

Grasp the ends of a rope (or the loop handles) attached to the low pulley of a cable apparatus with palms facing inward. Keep your feet shoulder-width apart, your torso erect, your knees slightly bent, and your core tight. Allow your arms to hang down from your shoulders in front of your body, but don't lock your elbows.

MOVEMENT

Pull the rope or handles up along the line of your body until your upper arms approach shoulder level. Keep your elbows higher than your wrists at all times. Contract your delts and lower the rope or handles along the same path back to the start position.

EXPERT TIPS

- Initiate the action by lifting the elbows, not the wrists, to ensure optimal stimulation of the target muscles.
- Be careful not to lift your elbows beyond a position that is parallel to the floor. Doing so can lead to shoulder impingement, which injures the rotator cuff.
- Keep your hands as close to your body as possible throughout the entire move.
- You can perform the move with a straight bar if you desire.

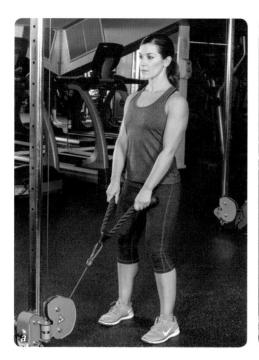 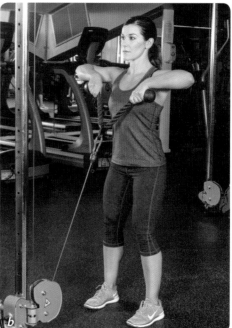

DUMBBELL LATERAL RAISE

This move targets the middle deltoids.

Shoulder Category 2

START

Sit at the edge of a flat bench or chair. Grasp two dumbbells and allow them to hang by your hips.

MOVEMENT

With a slight bend to your elbows, raise the dumbbells up and out to the sides until they reach shoulder level. At the top of the movement, the rear of the dumbbells should be slightly higher than the front (inward rotation of the shoulder). Contract your deltoids and return the weights along the same path to the start position.

EXPERT TIPS

- Think of pouring a cup of milk as you lift. This will keep maximal tension on the middle deltoids.
- This move can also be done standing.

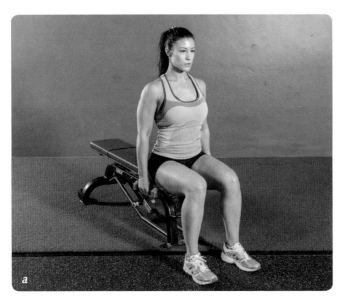
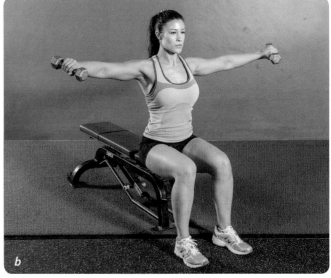

CABLE LATERAL RAISE

This move targets the middle deltoids.

Shoulder Category 2

START

Grasp a loop handle attached to the low pulley of a cable apparatus with your left hand. Stand so that your right side is facing the pulley, with your feet approximately shoulder-width apart, your torso erect, your knees slightly bent, and your core tight.

MOVEMENT

Maintain a slight bend to your elbow throughout the movement. Raise the handle across your body, up, and out to the side until it reaches the level of your shoulder. Contract your delts at the top of the movement and return the handle to the start position. After completing the desired number of reps, repeat the process on your right side.

EXPERT TIPS

- Think of pouring a cup of milk as you lift. Your pinky should be higher than your thumb at the top of the move; this keeps maximal tension on the middle deltoids.
- Keep your upper arms directly out to the sides at all times. Allowing them to gravitate inward switches the emphasis to the front delts at the expense of the middle delts.

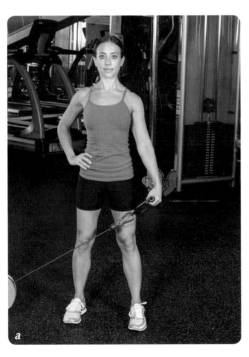
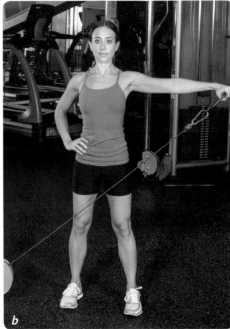

MACHINE LATERAL RAISE

This move targets the middle deltoids.

Shoulder Category 2

START

Sit in a lateral raise machine with your torso pressed to the pad. The seat should be adjusted so that your forearms align with the side pads. Place your forearms on the side pads, firmly grasping the attached handles with your palms facing each other.

MOVEMENT

Keeping your elbows flared, raise your upper arms up and out to the sides until they reach shoulder level. Contract your deltoids and return along the same path to the start position.

EXPERT TIP

Raise the weight only up to shoulder level; going higher than this can cause shoulder impingement.

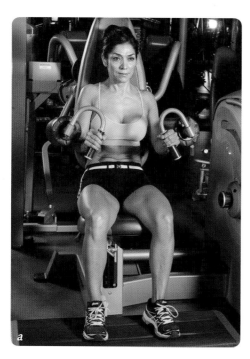
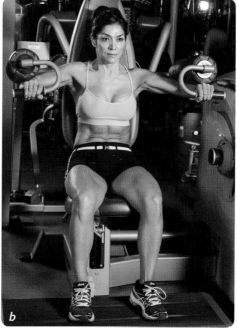

DUMBBELL SEATED BENT REVERSE FLY

This move targets the posterior (rear) deltoids. I prefer this to the standing version because it decreases stress to the low back.

Shoulder Category 3

START

Grasp two dumbbells and sit at the edge of a bench or chair. Bend your torso forward so that it is almost parallel to the floor. Allow the dumbbells to hang down in front of your body, palms facing each other.

MOVEMENT

With a slight bend to your elbows, raise the dumbbells up and out to the sides until they are parallel to the floor. Contract your delts at the top of the movement and return the dumbbells to the start position.

EXPERT TIPS

- Don't swing your body to complete a rep; this takes work away from the target muscles.
- There's a natural tendency to bring the elbows in toward the body while lifting. Avoid this tendency. The elbows should remain out away from your body throughout the move to keep tension on the rear delts.

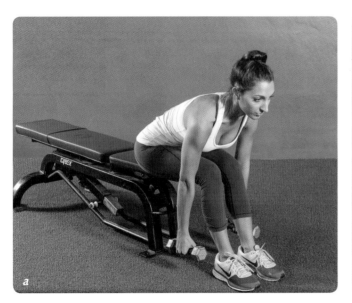
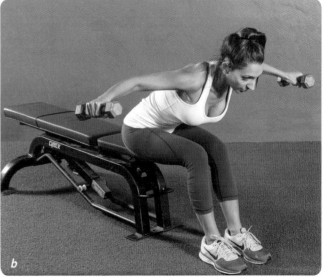

CABLE REVERSE FLY

This move targets the posterior delts.

Shoulder Category 3

START

Assume a shoulder-width stance in front of a cable-pulley apparatus. Grasp the end of the left cable with your right hand, and grasp the end of the right cable with your left hand. Keeping your torso rigid, take a couple of steps back to create tension in the pulleys.

MOVEMENT

Maintaining a slight bend to your arms, simultaneously pull the cables outward as far as comfortably possible in a circular direction. Contract your posterior deltoids and return to the start position.

EXPERT TIPS

- Do not straighten your arms as you perform the move. This causes the triceps to assist in the movement.
- Don't swing your body to complete a rep; this takes work away from the target muscles.

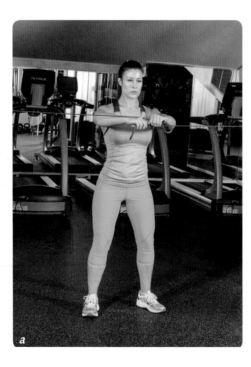
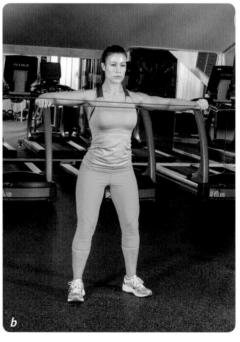

CABLE KNEELING BENT REVERSE FLY

This move targets the posterior (rear) deltoids.

Shoulder Category 3

START

Grasp a loop handle attached to the low pulley of a cable apparatus with your left hand and kneel down on your hands and knees. Stabilize your torso with your right arm. Position your left arm by your side with your elbow slightly bent.

MOVEMENT

Maintain a slight bend to your elbow and a tight core throughout the movement. Raise the handle out to your left side until your arm is parallel to the floor. Contract your delts at the top of the movement and return the handle to the start position. After completing the desired number of reps, repeat the process on your right side.

EXPERT TIP

Avoid the tendency to bring your elbows in toward your body as you lift. Your elbows should remain away from your body throughout the move to keep tension on your rear delts.

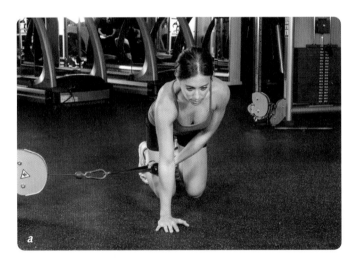
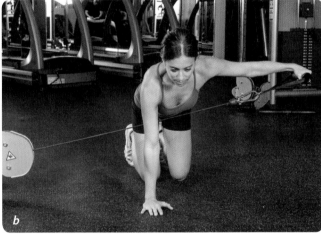

MACHINE REAR DELTOID FLY

This move targets the posterior (rear) deltoids.

Shoulder Category 3

START

Sit face-forward in a pec deck apparatus. With a slight bend to your elbows, grasp the machine handles with your palms facing each other or facing down.

MOVEMENT

Pull the handles back in a semicircular arc as far as comfortably possible, keeping your arms parallel to the floor at all times. Contract your rear delts and reverse direction, returning the handles to the start position.

EXPERT TIP

Your arms should remain parallel to the floor throughout the move. If they are not, adjust the seat height accordingly.

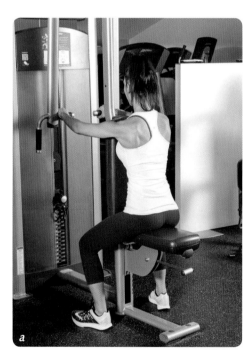 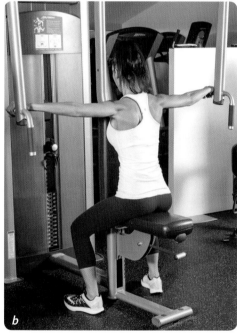

ELBOW FLEXOR EXERCISES

Exercises for the elbow flexors (biceps brachii, brachialis, brachioradialis) are divided into the following three categories (see table 3.2):

- Category 1 comprises exercises carried out with your arms at your sides or behind your body.
- Category 2 comprises exercises carried out with your arms in front of your body or raised to your sides.
- Category 3 comprises exercises carried out with your hands either pronated or in a neutral position.

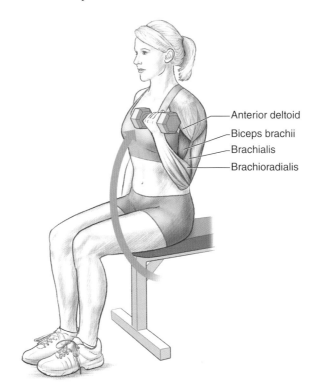

Anterior deltoid
Biceps brachii
Brachialis
Brachioradialis

Table 3.2 Elbow Flexor Exercises by Category

Category 1	Category 2	Category 3
Dumbbell biceps curl	Dumbbell preacher curl	Cable rope hammer curl
Dumbbell incline biceps curl	Concentration curl	Dumbbell hammer curl
Barbell drag curl	Dumbbell prone incline curl	Barbell reverse curl
Barbell curl	High-pulley cable curl	
Cable curl	Barbell preacher curl	

DUMBBELL BICEPS CURL

This move targets the biceps.

Elbow Flexor Category 1

START

Sit at the edge of a flat bench. Grasp a pair of dumbbells and allow them to hang at your sides with your palms facing forward.

MOVEMENT

Press your elbows into your sides and keep them stable throughout the move. Curl the dumbbells up toward your shoulders, and contract your biceps at the top of the move. Reverse direction and return to the start position.

EXPERT TIPS

- If desired, you can begin with your palms facing your sides and actively supinate your hands (turn your palms up) as you lift.
- Keep your wrists straight as you lift; roll them to complete the move.
- You can also perform this move standing.

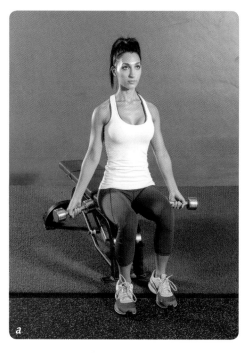
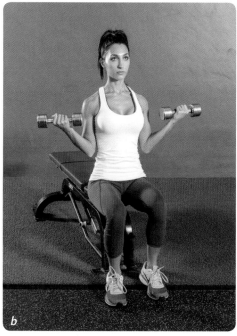

DUMBBELL INCLINE BICEPS CURL

This move targets the biceps. Because the arms are kept backward, it's especially effective for targeting the long head of the biceps.

Elbow Flexor Category 1

START

Lie supine (on your back) on a 40-degree incline bench. Grasp two dumbbells and allow the weights to hang behind your body with your palms facing forward.

MOVEMENT

Keeping your upper arms stable, curl the dumbbells up toward your shoulders. Contract your biceps; then return the weights to the start position.

EXPERT TIPS

- Make sure that your elbows stay back throughout the movement. This keeps maximal tension on the biceps, especially the long head.
- Keep your wrists straight as you lift; don't roll them to complete the move.
- You can alternate repetitions between your right and left arms, which may help you better focus on the individual target muscles.

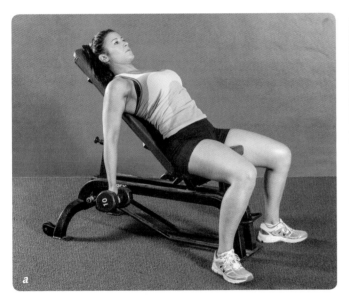 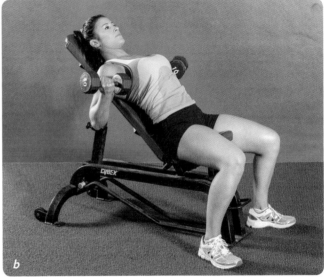

BARBELL DRAG CURL

This move targets the biceps, with an emphasis on the long head.

Elbow Flexor Category 1

START

Grasp a barbell with a palms-up, shoulder-width grip, and allow it to hang in front of your body with a slight bend to your elbows. Assume a comfortable stance and maintain a slight bend to your knees.

MOVEMENT

Keeping your upper arms close to your sides and stable throughout the move, bring your elbows back behind your body, curling the bar along the line of your torso up toward your shoulders. Contract your biceps and then reverse direction to return to the start position.

EXPERT TIP

Your elbows should move back as you lift; this keeps maximal tension on the long head.

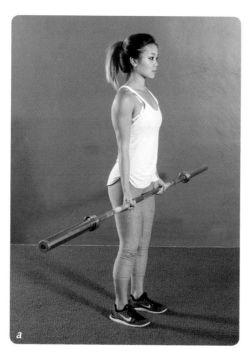
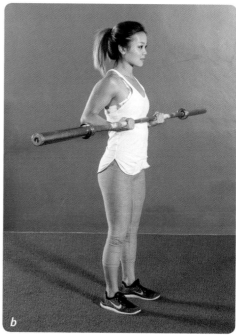

BARBELL CURL

This move targets the biceps.

Elbow Flexor Category 1

START

Assume a comfortable stance with a slight bend to your knees. Grasp a barbell with a palms-up, shoulder-width grip.

MOVEMENT

Keeping your upper arms pressed into your sides, curl the bar up toward your shoulders and contract your biceps at the top of the move. Reverse direction and return to the start position.

EXPERT TIPS

* Keep your upper arms motionless throughout the move; all activity takes place at the elbow.
* The move can be performed either with a straight bar or an EZ-Curl bar. The EZ-Curl bar can help to alleviate pressure on your wrists.

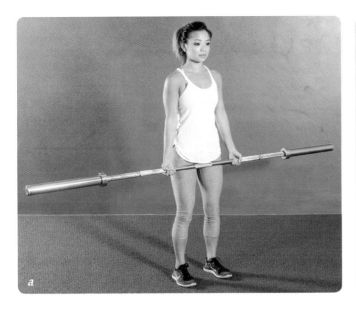
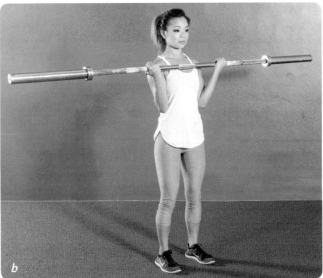

CABLE CURL

This move targets the biceps.

Elbow Flexor Category 1

START

Grasp a straight bar attached to the low pulley of a cable apparatus. Press your elbows into your sides, with your palms facing up. Keep your feet shoulder-width apart, your torso erect, your knees slightly bent, and your core tight.

MOVEMENT

Keeping your upper arms stable throughout the move, curl the bar up toward your shoulders. Contract your biceps, reverse the direction, and return to the start position.

EXPERT TIPS

- Keep your wrists straight as you lift; don't roll your wrists!
- Don't allow your upper arms to move forward as you lift. Doing so brings your shoulders into the movement at the expense of your arm muscles.
- You can train each arm separately by performing the movement with a loop handle.

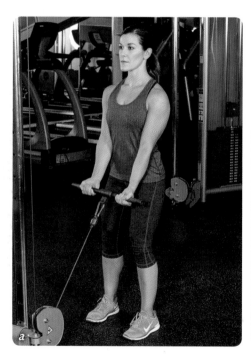 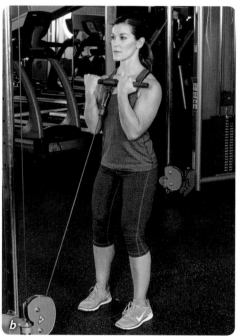

DUMBBELL PREACHER CURL

This move targets the biceps, with an emphasis on the short head.

Elbow Flexor Category 2

START

Grasp a dumbbell with your right hand. Place the upper portion of your right arm on a preacher curl unit or an incline bench, and allow your right forearm to extend just short of locking out the elbow.

MOVEMENT

Keeping your upper arm pressed to the bench, curl the dumbbell up toward your shoulder. Contract your biceps and then return the weight to the start position. After completing the desired number of reps, repeat on your left.

EXPERT TIPS

- Your upper arm should be fully braced on the bench. There should be no space between your arm and the bench.
- Keep your wrist straight as you lift; don't roll it to complete the move.

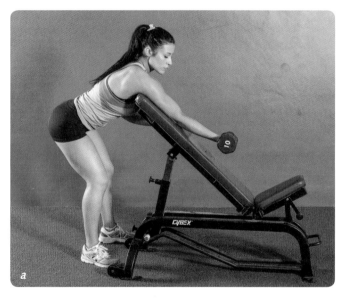
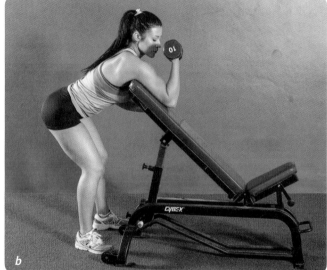

CONCENTRATION CURL

This move targets the biceps, with an emphasis on the short head.

Elbow Flexor Category 2

START

Sit at the edge of a flat bench with your legs wide apart. Grasp a dumbbell in your right hand, and brace your right triceps on the inside of your right thigh. Straighten your arm so that it hangs down near the floor.

MOVEMENT

Curl the weight up and in along the line of your body, contracting your biceps at the top of the move. Reverse direction and return to the start position. After completing the desired number of reps, repeat the process on your left.

EXPERT TIPS

- Keep your exercising arm braced to your inner thigh at all times. If you are struggling to complete a rep, use your opposite hand to assist the move rather than swinging your exercising arm.
- Keep your wrist straight as you lift; don't roll it to complete the move.

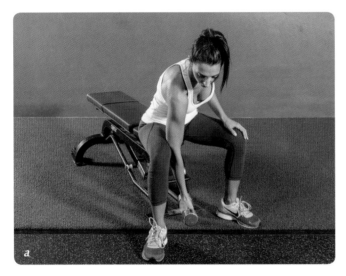
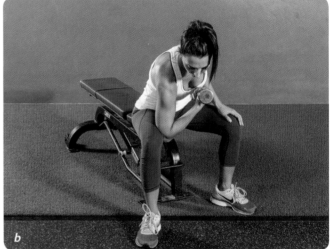

DUMBBELL PRONE INCLINE CURL

This move targets the biceps. Because the arms are held forward of the body, it's especially effective for targeting the short head.

Elbow Flexor Category 2

START

Lie prone (facedown) on an incline bench set at an approximately 30-degree angle. Grasp two dumbbells and allow the weights to hang straight down from your shoulders with your palms facing away from your body.

MOVEMENT

Curl the dumbbells up toward your shoulders, keeping your upper arms stable throughout the movement. Contract your biceps and then return the weights to the start position.

EXPERT TIPS

- Don't swing your arms as you lift. Doing so introduces unwanted momentum into the movement and reduces stress to the target muscles.
- Keep your wrists straight as you lift; don't roll them to complete the move.

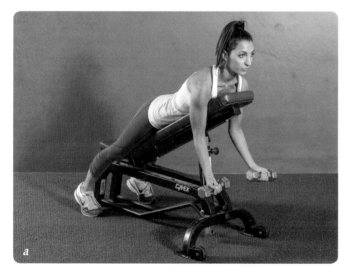

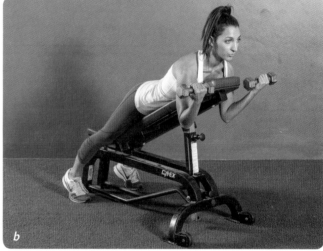

HIGH-PULLEY CABLE CURL

This move targets the biceps, particularly the short head.

Elbow Flexor Category 2

START

Grasp the loop handles of a high-pulley apparatus. Stand midway between the pulleys and allow your arms to extend just short of locking out the elbows. Your palms should face upward, and your low back should be slightly arched.

MOVEMENT

Keeping your upper arms fixed, curl the handles toward your shoulders. Contract your biceps; then return the handles to the start position.

EXPERT TIP

Don't allow your elbows to move forward during the move—this allows the long head of the biceps to exert greater force, thus diminishing stress to the short head, which is the target muscle of this exercise.

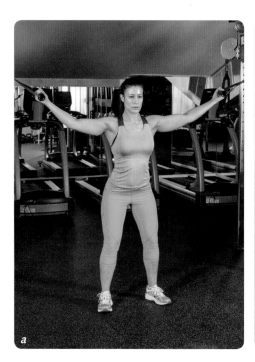
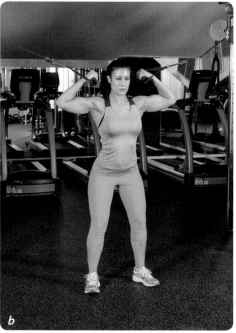

BARBELL PREACHER CURL

This move targets the biceps, with an emphasis on the short head.

Elbow Flexor Category 2

START

Grasp a barbell with both hands, palms turned up. Place the upper portion of your arms on the pad of a preacher curl bench, and allow your forearms to extend just short of locking out the elbow.

MOVEMENT

Keeping your upper arms pressed to the bench, curl the bar up toward your shoulders. Contract your biceps and then return the bar to the start position.

EXPERT TIPS

* Your upper arms should be fully braced on the pad. There should be no space between your arms and the bench.
* Keep your wrists straight as you lift; don't roll them to complete the move.

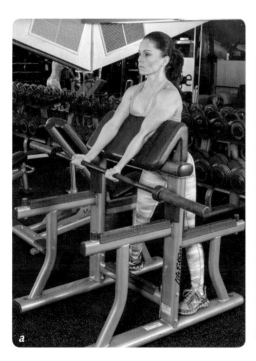
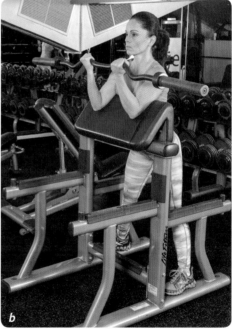

CABLE ROPE HAMMER CURL

This move targets the upper arms, with an emphasis on the brachialis.

Elbow Flexor Category 3

START

Grasp both ends of a rope (or loop handles) attached to the low pulley of a cable apparatus. Press your elbows into your sides with your palms facing each other. Keep your feet shoulder-width apart, your torso erect, your knees slightly bent, and your core tight.

MOVEMENT

Keeping your arms stable throughout the move, curl the rope up toward your shoulders and contract your biceps at the top of the move. Reverse the direction to return to the start position.

EXPERT TIPS

- Don't allow your upper arms to move forward as you lift. Doing so brings your shoulders into the movement at the expense of your arm muscles.
- Keep your wrists straight as you lift; don't roll them to complete the move.

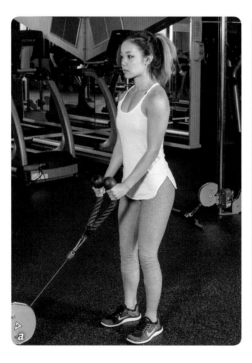 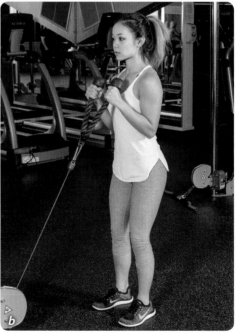

DUMBBELL HAMMER CURL

This move targets the upper arms, with an emphasis on the brachialis.

Elbow Flexor Category 3

START

Sit at the edge of a flat bench. Grasp a pair of dumbbells and allow them to hang at your sides with your palms facing each other.

MOVEMENT

Keeping your elbows pressed into your sides, curl the dumbbells up toward your shoulders while maintaining a neutral grip and contract your biceps at the top of the move. Reverse direction and return to the start position.

EXPERT TIP

Keep your wrists straight as you lift; don't roll them to complete the move.

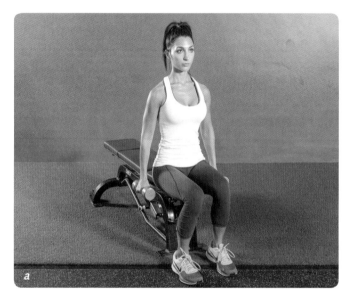
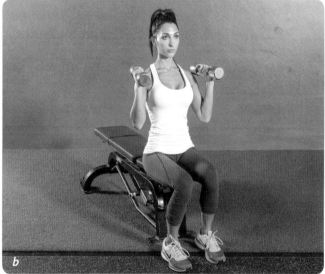

BARBELL REVERSE CURL

This move targets the brachialis.

Elbow Flexor Category 3

START

Assume a comfortable stance with a slight bend to your knees. Grasp a barbell with a palms-down, shoulder-width grip.

MOVEMENT

Keeping your upper arms pressed into your sides, curl the bar up toward your shoulders. Contract your elbow flexors at the top of the move and then return to the start position.

EXPERT TIPS

- Keep your upper arms motionless throughout the move. All activity takes place at the elbow.
- The move can be performed either with a straight bar or an EZ-Curl bar. The EZ-Curl bar can help to alleviate pressure on your wrists.

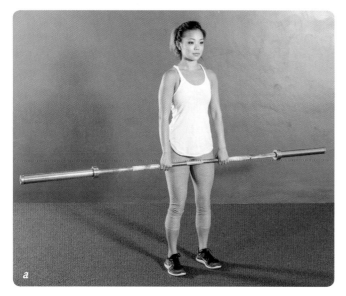
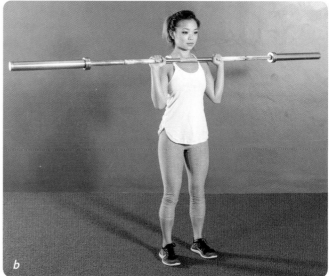

ELBOW EXTENSOR EXERCISES

Exercises for the elbow extensors (triceps brachii) are divided into the following three categories (see table 3.3):

- Category 1 comprises exercises carried out with your arms overhead.
- Category 2 comprises exercises carried out with your arms at your sides.
- Category 3 comprises exercises carried out with your arms midway between overhead and at your sides.

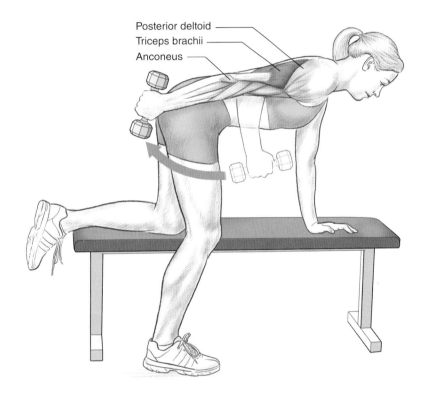

Table 3.3 Elbow Extensor Exercises by Category

Category 1	Category 2	Category 3
Cable rope overhead triceps extension	Cable triceps press-down	Skull crusher
Dumbbell overhead triceps extension	Cable triceps kickback	Dumbbell lying triceps extension
Machine overhead triceps extension	Triceps dip	Close-grip bench press
	Dumbbell triceps kickback	

CABLE ROPE OVERHEAD TRICEPS EXTENSION

This move targets the triceps, particularly the long head of the muscle.

Elbow Extensor Category 1

START

Grasp the ends of a rope (or loop handles) attached to the low pulley of a cable apparatus and turn your body away from the pulley. Bring your elbows up close to your ears, bend your elbows, and allow your hands to hang down behind your head as far as comfortably possible, with your palms facing each other. Bring one foot in front of the other, with your torso erect and your knees slightly bent.

MOVEMENT

Keeping your elbows close to your ears, straighten your arms as fully as possible. Contract your triceps and then lower the weight along the same path back to the start position.

EXPERT TIPS

- Make sure that your elbows stay pinned to your ears as you lift. Flared elbows will reduce stress to the triceps.
- Your upper arms should remain completely stationary throughout the move. Any forward movement diminishes tension on the triceps.
- If you desire, you can perform this exercise one arm at a time. This may alleviate stress on your elbows and help you focus on each arm individually.

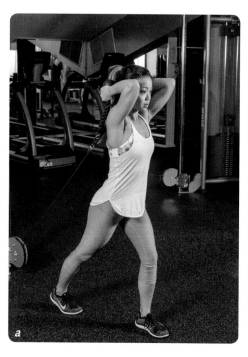 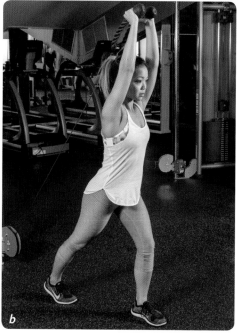

DUMBBELL OVERHEAD TRICEPS EXTENSION

This move targets the triceps, particularly the long head.

Elbow Extensor Category 1

START

Grasp the stem of a dumbbell with one hand. Sit at the edge of a flat bench or chair, bring the dumbbell overhead, bend your elbow, and allow the weight to hang down behind your head as far as comfortably possible.

MOVEMENT

Straighten your arm upward, keeping your elbow back and pointed toward the ceiling throughout the move. Contract your triceps and then lower the weight along the same path back to the start position.

EXPERT TIPS

- Keep your elbow pinned to your ear as you lift. Flared elbows will reduce stress to the triceps.
- If you have difficulty maintaining an erect posture, place the bench in the upright position and brace your back against the pad.
- Performing this exercise one arm at a time may alleviate stress on your elbows as well as allow you to focus on each arm individually.

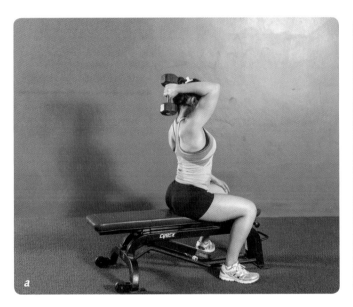
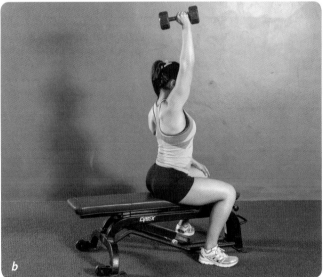

MACHINE OVERHEAD TRICEPS EXTENSION

This move targets the triceps, particularly the long head of the muscle.

Elbow Extensor Category 1

START

Sit upright in an overhead triceps machine, press your back against the seat pad, and grasp the machine handles. Press your elbows close to your ears if the machine allows, bend your elbows, and allow your hands to hang down behind your head as far as comfortably possible.

MOVEMENT

Keeping your elbows close to your ears, straighten your arms as fully as possible. Contract your triceps and then lower the weight along the same path to the start position.

EXPERT TIPS

- Make sure that your elbows stay pinned to your ears as you lift. Flared elbows will reduce stress to the triceps.
- Your upper arms should remain completely stationary throughout the move. Any forward movement diminishes tension on the triceps.

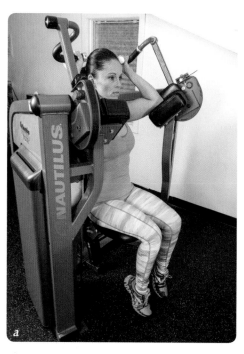
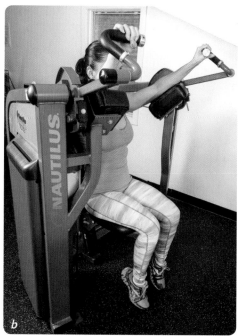

CABLE TRICEPS PRESS-DOWN

This move targets the triceps, particularly the medial and lateral heads.

Elbow Extensor Category 2

START

Use an overhand grip to grasp the ends of a rope (or loop handles) attached to the high pulley of a cable apparatus. Keep your feet shoulder-width apart, your torso erect, your knees slightly bent, and your core tight. Press your upper arms against your sides with your elbows bent at a 90-degree angle and your palms facing each other.

MOVEMENT

Keeping your elbows at your sides, straighten your arms as far as possible without discomfort. Contract your triceps, reverse the direction, and return to the start position.

EXPERT TIPS

- Don't allow your arms to move out as you lift. Doing so brings the chest muscles into play at the expense of the triceps.
- For an added contraction, you can turn your palms out so that they face away from each other at the end of the move.
- The move can be done with a variety of attachments, including a curved bar, a straight bar, or loop handles.

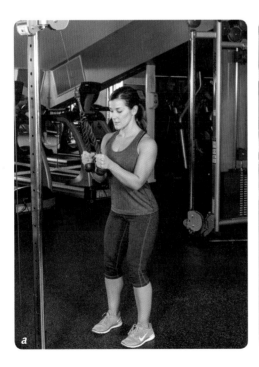
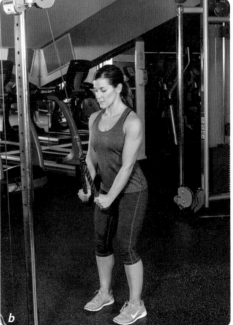

CABLE TRICEPS KICKBACK

This move targets the triceps, particularly the medial and lateral heads.

Elbow Extensor Category 2

START

Grasp a loop handle attached to the mid-pulley of a cable apparatus. Bend your torso forward so that it is at a 45-degree angle to the floor. Press your left arm against your side with your left elbow bent at a 90-degree angle and your palm facing backward. Keep your feet shoulder-width apart, your torso erect, and your knees slightly bent.

MOVEMENT

Keeping your upper arm stable, raise the handle by straightening your arm until it is parallel to the floor. Then, reverse the direction and return the weight to the start position. After performing the desired number of repetitions, repeat the process on your right side.

EXPERT TIPS

- Don't let your upper arm sag as you lift. This negatively affects tension to the target muscles.
- Don't flick your wrists at the top of movement. This a common performance error that fatigues the forearm muscles before the triceps and reduces the effectiveness of the move.
- Keep your back slightly arched throughout the movement. Never round your spine; doing so places undue stress on the lumbar area and could lead to injury.

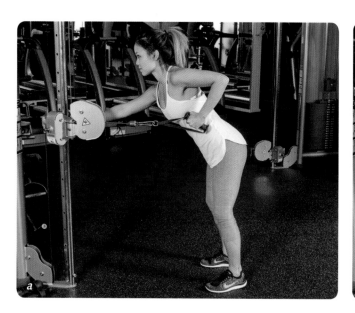 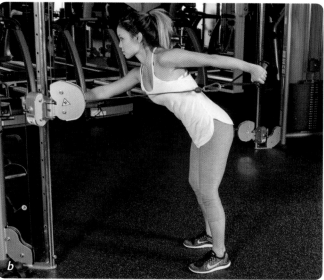

TRICEPS DIP

This move targets the triceps, particularly the medial and lateral heads.

Elbow Extensor Category 2

START

While sitting on a flat bench, place your heels on the floor with a slight bend to your knees and your palms on the edge of the flat bench, arms straight.

MOVEMENT

Bend your elbows as far as comfortably possible, allowing your butt to descend below the level of the bench. Make sure that your elbows stay close to your body throughout the move. Reverse direction by forcibly straightening your arms and return to the start position.

EXPERT TIPS

- You can make the move easier by bending more at the knees, or make it harder by reducing your knee bend and extending your feet farther outward.
- Keep your back close to the bench at all times. If your body gravitates forward, you place increased stress on the shoulder joint.

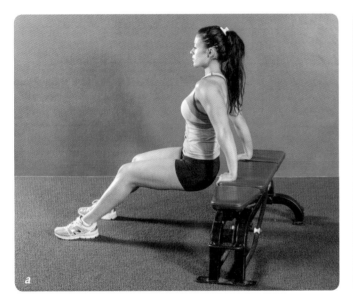
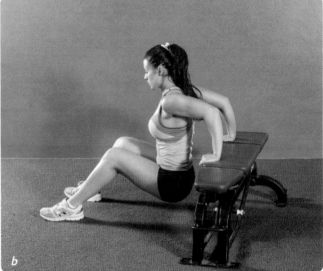

DUMBBELL TRICEPS KICKBACK

This move targets the triceps, particularly the medial and lateral heads.

Elbow Extensor Category 2

START

Stand with your upper body bent forward so that it is virtually parallel to the floor. Grasp a dumbbell with your right hand, and press your right arm against your side with your elbow bent at a 90-degree angle.

MOVEMENT

With your palm facing your body, raise the weight by straightening your arm until it is parallel to the floor. Then, reverse direction and return the weight to the start position. After performing the desired number of repetitions, repeat on your left.

EXPERT TIPS

- Don't let your upper arm sag down as you lift. Doing so reduces the effects of gravity and thus diminishes tension to the target muscles.
- Don't flick your wrist at the top of movement. This is a common error that fatigues the forearm muscles before the triceps and reduces the effectiveness of the move.

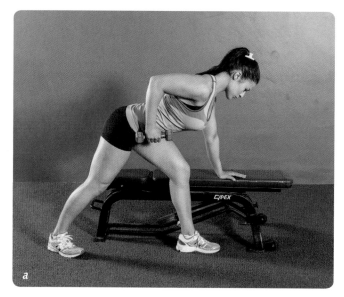
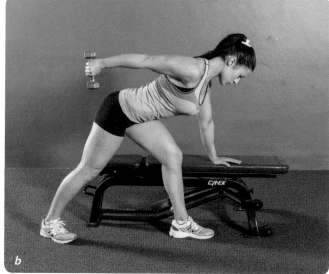

SKULL CRUSHER

This move is also called the nose breaker. Don't worry, though; as long as you use proper form, you won't break any bones! The target muscles are the triceps.

Elbow Extensor Category 3

START

Lie supine on a flat bench with your feet planted firmly on the floor. Grasp an EZ-Curl bar (or a barbell) with your palms facing away from your body, and straighten your arms so that the bar is directly over your chest (your arms should be perpendicular to your body).

MOVEMENT

Keeping your elbows in and pointed toward the ceiling, bend at the elbows to lower the bar until the bar is just above the level of your forehead. Press the bar back up until it reaches the start position.

EXPERT TIP

Keep your upper arms perpendicular to the floor at all times. This maintains roughly equal tension to all three triceps heads.

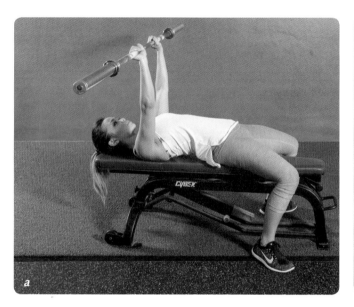 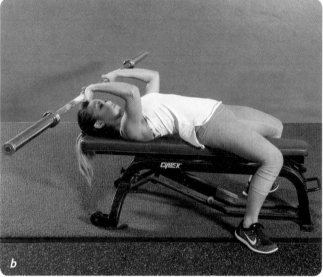

DUMBBELL LYING TRICEPS EXTENSION

This move targets the triceps.

Elbow Extensor Category 3

START

Lie supine on a flat bench with your feet planted firmly on the floor. Grasp a straight bar or a dumbbell in each hand and straighten your arms so that the dumbbells are directly over your chest (your arms should be perpendicular to your body).

MOVEMENT

Keeping your elbows in and pointed toward the ceiling, bend at the elbows to lower the dumbbells until they reach a point just above the level of your forehead. Press the dumbbells back up until they reach the start position.

EXPERT TIPS

- Keep your elbows aligned with your ears as you lift. Flared elbows will reduce the stress to the triceps.
- This exercise can also be performed one arm at a time, which allows you to focus on each arm individually.

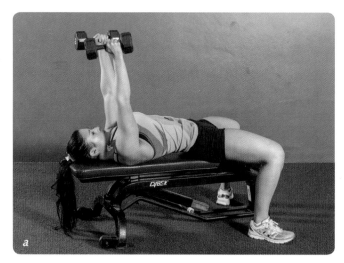
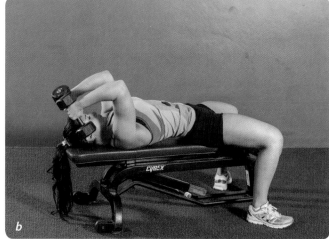

CLOSE-GRIP BENCH PRESS

This move targets the triceps. The pecs also are worked to a significant degree.

Elbow Extensor Category 3

START

Lie supine on a flat bench with your feet planted firmly on the floor. Grasp a straight bar or an EZ-Curl bar with your hands approximately 1 foot (30 cm) apart. Bend your elbows to bring the bar directly under your pecs.

MOVEMENT

Keeping your elbows close to your sides, press the weight straight up over your chest. Contract your triceps and return the bar along the same path to the start position.

EXPERT TIP

Don't grip the bar with your hands too close together. Doing so causes the elbows to flare, reducing stress to the triceps. The goal is to keep your elbows close to your sides at all times.

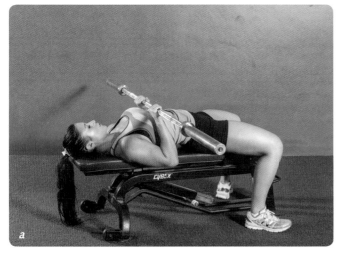
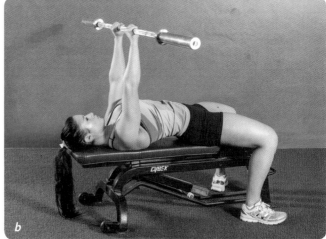

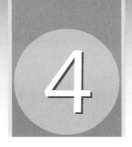

Exercises for the Lower Body

This chapter describes and illustrates exercises for the muscles of the lower body. Read the descriptions carefully, and scrutinize the photos to ensure proper form. I have provided expert tips for each of these movements to optimize your training performance. Remember that exercises are merely tools, or a means to an end—in this case, for enhancing muscular development. If an exercise does not feel right to you, simply substitute it for a comparable move.

FRONTAL THIGH AND HIP EXERCISES

Exercises for the frontal thighs and hips are divided into the following three categories (see table 4.1):

- Category 1 comprises multijoint bilateral (both legs at the same time) lower-body exercises.
- Category 2 comprises multijoint unilateral (one leg at a time) lower-body exercises.
- Category 3 comprises single-joint lower-body exercises targeting the quadriceps.

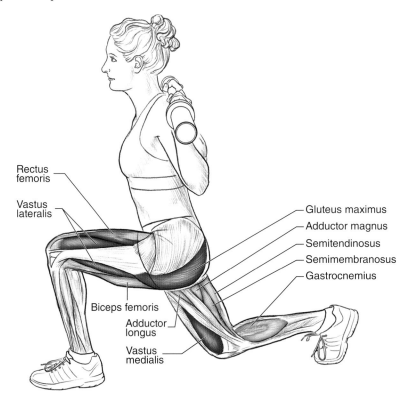

Table 4.1 Frontal Thigh and Hip Exercises by Category

Category 1	Category 2	Category 3
Deadlift	Bulgarian split squat	Leg extension
Barbell back squat	Dumbbell lunge	Single-leg extension
Barbell front squat	Dumbbell reverse lunge	Sissy squat
Goblet squat	Dumbbell side lunge	
Leg press	Dumbbell step-up	
	Barbell lunge	
	Barbell reverse lunge	
	Barbell split squat	

DEADLIFT

This move targets the entire lower-body musculature while also working many of the upper-body muscles.

Frontal Thigh and Hip Category 1

START

Assume a shoulder-width stance a few inches (about 7 cm) in front of a barbell that rests on the floor. Bend your knees and grasp the bar with an alternating grip (one hand over the bar, the other under the bar), with your hands just outside of your legs. Your spine should be in a neutral position.

MOVEMENT

Keeping your head up, chest out, and arms straight, drive the weight upward by forcefully extending your legs and hips. As you reach the top of the lift, contract your glutes, and then return to the start position.

EXPERT TIPS

- Keep your shins as close to the bar as possible when you lift. This maximizes leverage for the movement.
- Do not hyperextend your low back at the top of the lift. Rather, your body should form a straight line as you contract your glutes.
- Lifting straps can be used if you have trouble holding the weight.

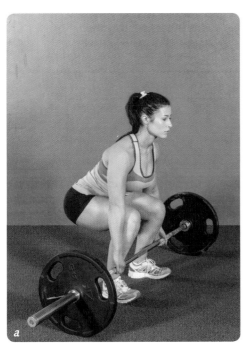
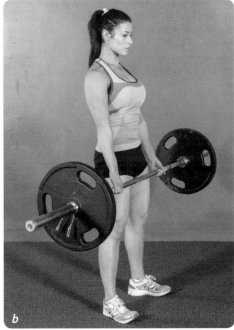

BARBELL BACK SQUAT

This move targets the thighs and glutes, with secondary emphasis on the hamstrings. It is the quintessential lower-body exercise and one of the most functional movements you can perform, activating over 200 muscles in the body.

Frontal Thigh and Hip Category 1

START

Rest a straight bar high on the back of your neck, grasping the bar with both hands at a width that allows your arms to form right angles. Assume a shoulder-width stance with your feet turned slightly outward.

MOVEMENT

Keeping your core muscles tight, lower your body until your thighs are parallel to the floor. Your low back should be slightly arched, and your heels should stay in contact with the floor at all times. When you reach a seated position, reverse direction by straightening your legs and return to the start position.

EXPERT TIPS

- Your knees should travel in the same plane as your toes at all times.
- Your heels should stay in contact with the floor at all times. If you have trouble keeping your heels down, place a 1-inch (2.5 cm) block of wood or a weight plate underneath them.
- Wrap a towel around the bar if it feels uncomfortable on your neck.

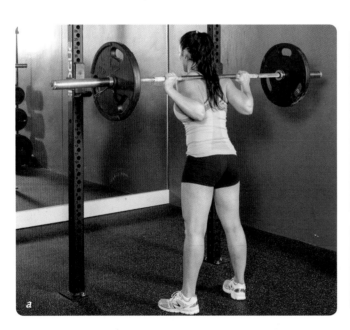
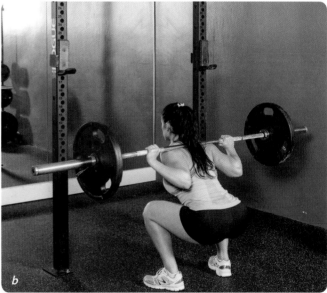

BARBELL FRONT SQUAT

This is a great movement for targeting the frontal thighs while minimizing activation of the glutes.

Frontal Thigh and Hip Category 1

START

Rest a straight bar across your upper chest, holding it in place with both hands. Assume a shoulder-width stance with your feet turned slightly outward, your shoulders back, and your chin up.

MOVEMENT

Keeping your core muscles tight, lower your body until your thighs are parallel to the floor. Your low back should be slightly arched, and your heels should stay in contact with the floor at all times. When you reach a seated position, reverse direction by straightening your legs and return to the start position.

EXPERT TIPS

- Your knees should travel in the same plane as your toes at all times.
- Your heels should stay in contact with the floor at all times. If you have trouble keeping your heels down, place a 1-inch (2.5 cm) block of wood or a weight plate underneath them.
- Wrap a towel around the bar if it feels uncomfortable on your chest.

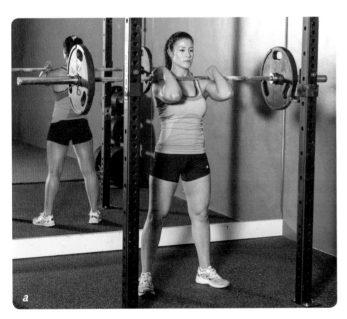
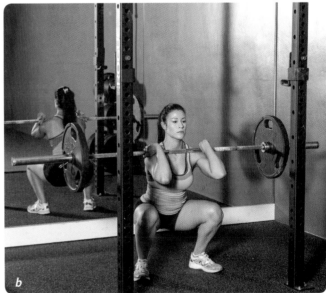

GOBLET SQUAT

This move targets the thighs and glutes.

Frontal Thigh and Hip Category 1

START

Hold the top of a dumbbell with both hands and bring it to rest at the top of your chest. Assume a shoulder-width stance with your feet turned slightly outward, your shoulders back, and your chin up.

MOVEMENT

Keeping your core muscles tight and the dumbbell pressed to your upper chest, lower your body until your thighs are parallel to the floor. Your low back should be slightly arched, and your heels should stay in contact with the floor at all times. When you reach a seated position, reverse direction by straightening your legs and returning to the start position.

EXPERT TIPS

- Your knees should travel in the same plane as your toes at all times.
- Your heels should stay in contact with the floor at all times. If you have trouble keeping your heels down, place a 1-inch (2.5 cm) block of wood or a weight plate underneath them.

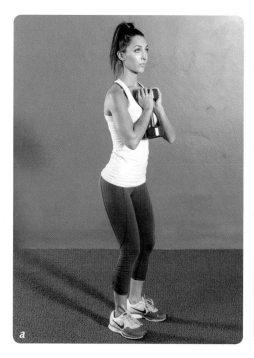
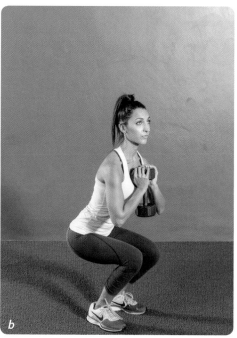

LEG PRESS

This move targets the glutes and the quads, with secondary emphasis on the hamstrings.

Frontal Thigh and Hip Category 1

START

Sit upright in a leg press unit, pressing your back firmly against the padded seat. Place your feet on the footplate with a shoulder-width stance. Straighten your legs with your toes angled slightly outward, and unlock the carriage-release bars located on the sides of the machine.

MOVEMENT

Keeping your back pressed firmly against the padded seat, lower your legs, bringing your knees in toward your chest. Without bouncing at the bottom, press the weight up in a controlled fashion and contract your quads, stopping just before you lock your knees.

EXPERT TIP

Placing your feet high on the footplate increases stimulation of the glutes; keeping your feet low emphasizes the quads.

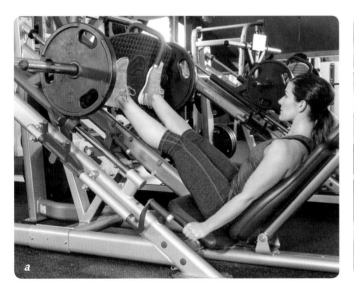
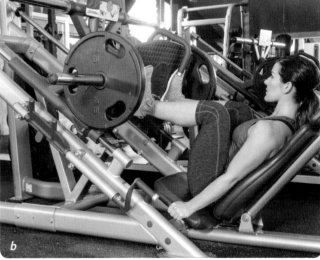

BULGARIAN SPLIT SQUAT

This move targets the quads and glutes. Secondary emphasis is on the hamstrings. This is an excellent move to promote the independent development of each leg and to correct muscle imbalances between the thighs.

Frontal Thigh and Hip Category 2

START

Grasp two dumbbells and allow your arms to hang down by your sides with your palms facing your body. Stand approximately 2 feet (60 cm) in front of a raised object (e.g., bench, step, chair), facing away from it, and place your left instep on top of the object behind you. Your back should be straight, your head up, and your chest out.

MOVEMENT

Keeping your right foot flat on the floor, lower your body until your right thigh is approximately parallel to the floor. Your low back should be slightly arched, and your right heel should stay in contact with the floor at all times. When you reach a seated position, reverse direction by straightening your right leg and return to the start position. After performing the desired number of repetitions, repeat on the opposite side.

EXPERT TIPS

- You can increase the difficulty of the exercise by raising the bench height.
- Look upward as you perform the move; this helps to prevent rounding of the upper spine.

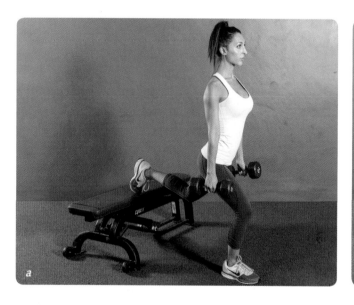 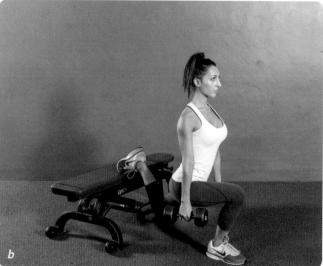

DUMBBELL LUNGE

This move targets the thighs and glutes.

Frontal Thigh and Hip Category 2

START

Grasp two dumbbells and allow them to hang down by your sides with your palms facing your body. Assume a shoulder-width stance with your shoulders back and your chin up.

MOVEMENT

Keeping your core muscles tight, take a long step forward with your left leg, lowering your body by flexing your left knee and hip. Continue your descent until your right knee is almost in contact with the floor. Reverse direction by forcibly extending the left hip and knee, bringing the leg back until you return to the start position. Perform the move the same way on your right; then alternate between legs until you have reached the desired number of repetitions.

EXPERT TIPS

- Make sure that your front knee travels in line with the plane of your toes.
- Focus on dropping down on your rear leg. This keeps the front knee from pushing too far forward, which can place undue stress on the joint capsule.
- Look upward as you perform the move; this helps to prevent rounding of the upper spine.

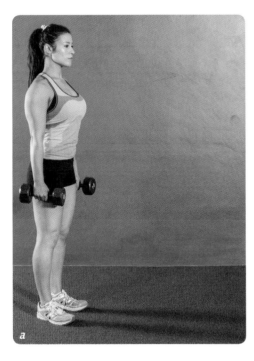 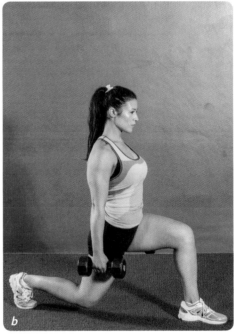

DUMBBELL REVERSE LUNGE

This move targets most of the lower-body muscles, with particular emphasis on the quads and glutes. It's an excellent exercise for improving dynamic balance.

Frontal Thigh and Hip Category 2

START

Grasp two dumbbells and allow them to hang down by your sides with your palms facing your body. Assume a shoulder-width stance with your shoulders back and your chin up.

MOVEMENT

Keeping your core muscles tight, take a long step backward with your right leg, lowering your body by flexing your right knee and hip in the process. Continue your descent until your right knee is almost in contact with the floor. Reverse direction by forcibly extending the right hip and knee, bringing the leg forward until you return to the start position. Perform the move the same way on your left; then alternate between legs until you reach the desired number of repetitions.

EXPERT TIPS

- A longer stride emphasizes more of the glutes; a shorter stride targets the quads.
- Look upward as you perform the move; this helps to prevent rounding of the upper spine.

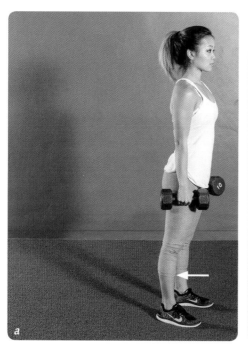
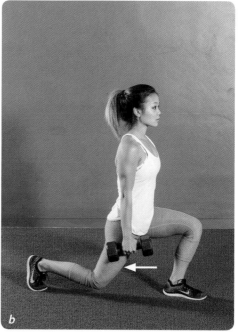

DUMBBELL SIDE LUNGE

This move targets the muscles of the lower body with a particular emphasis on the adductors of the inner thigh. It's a good exercise to promote lateral balance.

Frontal Thigh and Hip Category 2

START

Assume a wide stance, approximately 1 foot (30 cm) or more past shoulder width. Grasp two dumbbells and hold one in front and one in back of your body.

MOVEMENT

Keeping your left leg straight, bend your right knee out to the side until your right thigh is parallel to the floor. Forcefully rise back up and repeat this process immediately on your left; then alternate between legs until you reach the desired number of repetitions.

EXPERT TIPS

- Make sure that your front knee travels in line with the plane of your toes.
- Focus on dropping down on your straight leg. This keeps the bent knee from pushing too far forward, which can place undue stress on the joint capsule.
- Look upward as you perform the move; this helps to prevent rounding of the upper spine.

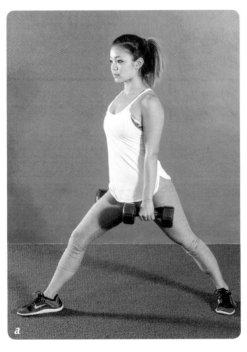
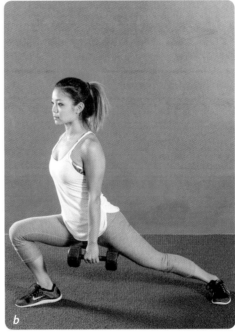

DUMBBELL STEP-UP

This move targets the thighs and glutes.

Frontal Thigh and Hip Category 2

START

Grasp a pair of dumbbells and allow them to hang at your sides with your palms facing your body. Stand facing the side of a flat bench with your feet shoulder-width apart.

MOVEMENT

Pushing off your left leg, step up with your right foot and follow with your left foot so that both feet are flat on the bench. Step back down in the same order, first with your right foot and then with your left, returning to the start position. Continue alternate stepping for the desired number of repetitions.

EXPERT TIPS

- A higher step increases stimulation of the glutes.
- Look upward as you perform the move; this helps to prevent rounding of the upper spine.

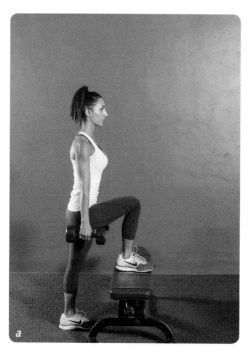
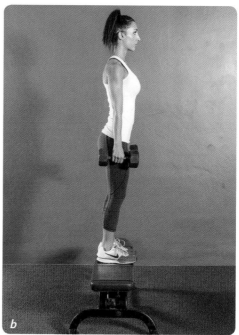

BARBELL LUNGE

This move targets the thighs and glutes. It's a good move for developing dynamic balance.

Frontal Thigh and Hip Category 2

START

Rest a barbell on your shoulders behind your neck, grasping the bar on both sides to maintain balance. Assume a shoulder-width stance with your shoulders back and your chin up.

MOVEMENT

Keeping your core tight, take a long step forward with your left leg, lowering your body by flexing your left knee and hip. Continue your descent until your right knee is almost in contact with the floor. Reverse direction by forcibly extending the left hip and knee, bringing the leg back until you return to the start position. Perform the move the same way on your right; then alternate between legs until you reach the desired number of repetitions.

EXPERT TIPS

- Make sure that your knee travels in line with the plane of your toes.
- Focus on dropping down on your rear leg. This keeps the front knee from pushing too far forward, which can place undue stress on the joint capsule.

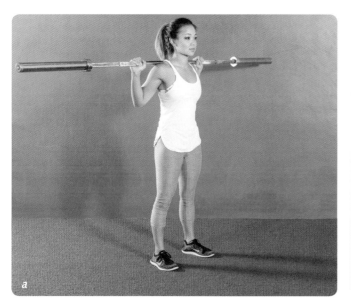

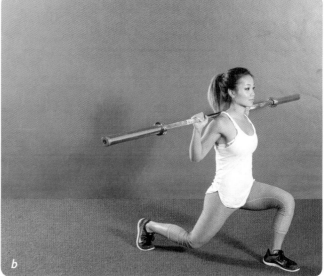

BARBELL REVERSE LUNGE

This move targets most of the lower-body muscles, with particular emphasis on the quads and glutes. It's an excellent exercise for improving dynamic balance.

Frontal Thigh and Hip Category 2

START

Place a barbell behind your neck and stabilize by grasping the bar with a grip slightly wider than shoulder width. Assume a shoulder-width stance with your shoulders back and your chin up.

MOVEMENT

Keeping your core muscles tight, take a long step backward with your right leg, lowering your body by flexing your right knee and hip. Continue your descent until your right knee is almost in contact with the floor. Reverse direction by forcibly extending the right hip and knee, bringing the leg forward until you return to the start position. Perform the move the same way on your left; then alternate between legs until you reach the desired number of repetitions.

EXPERT TIPS

- A longer stride emphasizes more of the glutes; a shorter stride targets the quads.
- Look upward as you perform the move; this helps to prevent rounding of the upper spine.

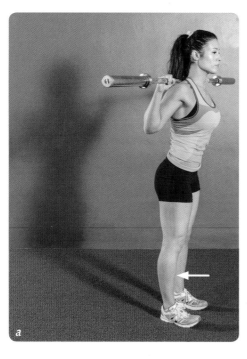
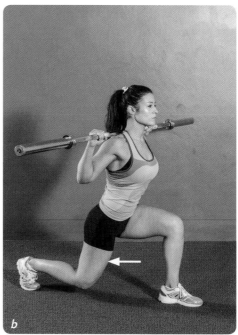

BARBELL SPLIT SQUAT

This move targets the thighs and glutes. It's a good move to develop static balance.

Frontal Thigh and Hip Category 2

START

Rest a barbell across your shoulders, grasping the bar on both sides to maintain balance. Take a long stride forward with your left leg, and raise your right heel so that your right foot is on its toes. Keep your shoulders back and your chin up.

MOVEMENT

Keeping your core muscles tight, lower your body by flexing your left knee and hip, continuing your descent until your right knee is almost in contact with the floor. Reverse direction by forcibly extending the left hip and knee until you return to the start position. After performing the desired number of reps, repeat the process on your right.

EXPERT TIPS

- Make sure that your knee travels in line with the plane of your toes.
- Focus on dropping down on your rear leg. This keeps the front knee from pushing too far forward, which can place undue stress on the joint capsule.

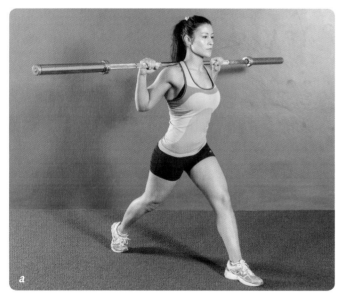
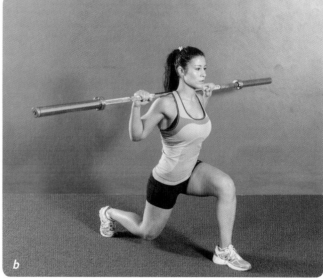

LEG EXTENSION

This move targets the quadriceps.

Frontal Thigh and Hip Category 3

START

Sit upright in a leg extension unit so that the undersides of your knees touch the edge of the seat. Bend your knees and place your insteps underneath the roller pad located at the bottom of the machine. Grasp the machine's handles for support, tighten your core muscles, and straighten your back.

MOVEMENT

Keeping your thighs and upper body immobile, lift your feet up until your legs are almost parallel to the floor. Contract your quads and then reverse the direction, returning to the start position.

EXPERT TIPS

- Because of the high shear forces associated with this move, it may not be suitable for those with knee problems. When in doubt, check with your physician.
- There is no tangible benefit to turning your feet in or out, and doing so can increase the risk of knee injury. Keep them pointed straight ahead.

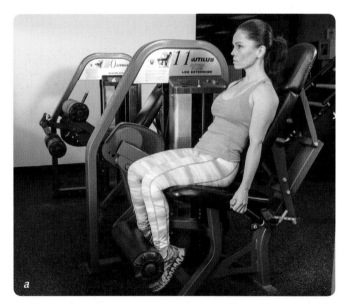
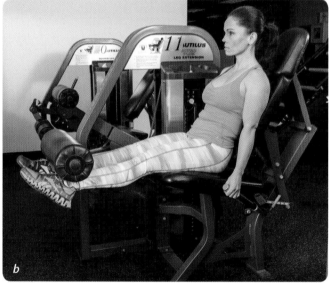

SINGLE-LEG EXTENSION

This move targets the quadriceps.

Frontal Thigh and Hip Category 3

START

Sit upright in a leg extension unit so that the undersides of your knees touch the edge of the seat. Bend your left knee and place your left instep underneath the roller pad located at the bottom of the machine. Keep your right leg back so that it is off the roller pad. Grasp the machine's handles for support, tighten your core, and straighten your back.

MOVEMENT

Keeping your thighs and upper body immobile, lift your left foot up until your left lower leg is almost parallel to the floor. Contract your quads and then reverse the direction, returning to the start position. After performing the desired number of reps, repeat the process on your right side.

EXPERT TIPS

- Because of the high shear forces associated with this move, it may not be suitable for those with knee problems. When in doubt, check with your physician.
- There is no tangible benefit to turning your feet in or out, and doing so can increase the risk of knee injury. Keep them pointed straight ahead.

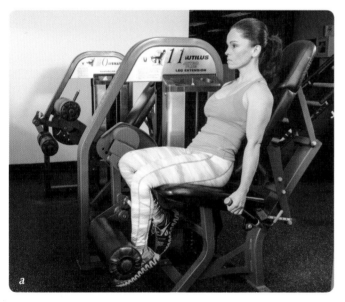
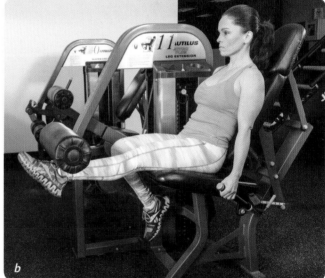

SISSY SQUAT

This move targets the quadriceps, with particular emphasis on the rectus femoris.

Frontal Thigh and Hip Category 3

START

Assume a shoulder-width stance. Grasp a stationary object with one hand and rise up onto your toes.

MOVEMENT

In one motion, slant your torso back, bend your knees, and lower your body. Thrust your knees forward as you descend, and lean back until your shins are almost parallel to the floor. Then, reverse direction and rise up until you reach the start position.

EXPERT TIPS

- Make sure that you remain on your toes throughout the move; keeping your feet planted can result in knee injury.
- If the exercise becomes too easy (i.e., you are not challenged within your given rep range), you can hold a dumbbell or weight plate to your chest for added intensity.
- This move may be contraindicated for those with existing knee injury.

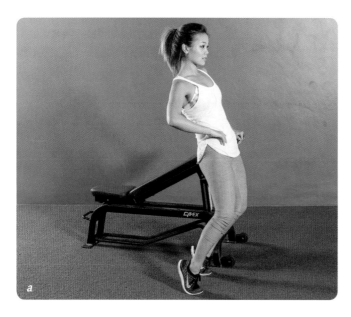
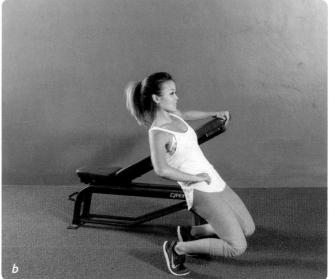

POSTERIOR THIGH AND HIP EXERCISES

Exercises for the posterior thighs and hips are divided into the following two categories (see table 4.2):

- Category 1 comprises single-joint exercises that target the glutes and hamstrings through hip extension or abduction.
- Category 2 comprises single-joint exercises that directly target the hamstrings through knee flexion.

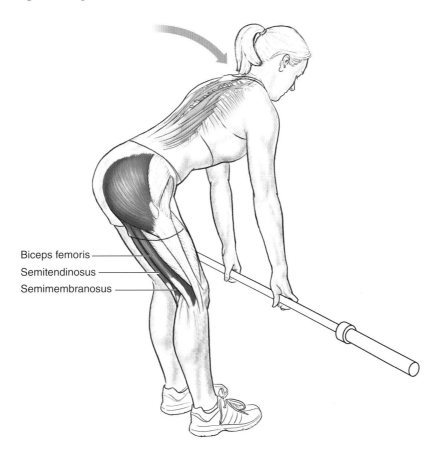

Biceps femoris
Semitendinosus
Semimembranosus

Table 4.2   Posterior Thigh and Hip Exercises by Category

Category 1	Category 2
Good morning	Lying leg curl
Barbell stiff-leg deadlift	Machine kneeling leg curl
Dumbbell stiff-leg deadlift	Machine seated leg curl
Barbell glute bridge	Stability ball leg curl
Barbell hip thrust	
Cable glute back kick	
Reverse hyperextension	
Hyperextension	
Cable standing abduction	

GOOD MORNING

This move targets the glutes and hamstrings.

Posterior Thigh and Hip Category 1

START

Rest a barbell across your shoulders, grasping the bar on both sides to maintain balance. Assume a shoulder-width stance with your head up and your knees and back straight.

MOVEMENT

Keeping your low back taut throughout the movement, bend forward at the hips until your upper body is roughly parallel to the floor. In a controlled fashion, reverse direction, contracting your glutes as you raise your body up along the same path back to the start position.

EXPERT TIPS

- Wrap a towel around the bar if it feels uncomfortable on your neck.
- Move only at the hips, not the waist! The action is purely hip extension; any spinal movement will place the vertebrae at risk of injury. The long moment arm in this movement makes a tight core of utmost importance.
- This move is not recommended for those with existing low back injury.

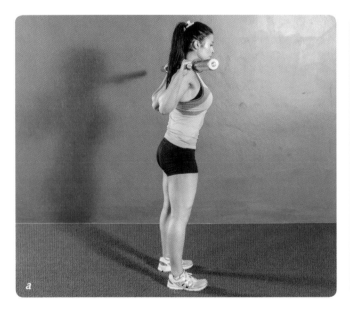
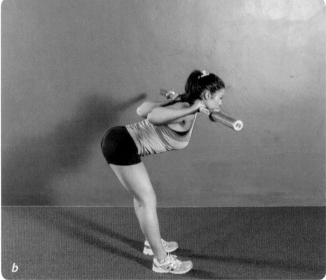

BARBELL STIFF-LEG DEADLIFT

This move targets the glutes and hamstrings.

Posterior Thigh and Hip Category 1

START

Stand with your feet shoulder-width apart. Grasp a straight bar and let it hang in front of your body.

MOVEMENT

Keeping your knees straight, bend forward at the hips and lower the barbell until you feel an intense stretch in your hamstrings. Then, reverse direction, contracting your glutes as you rise up to the start position.

EXPERT TIPS

- You should bend forward only at the hips, not the low back. The action is purely hip extension; any spinal movement will place the vertebrae at risk of injury.
- There is rarely a need to stand on a box, as many people do. This is necessary only if you can touch your toes without flexing your spine—a feat very few can do.

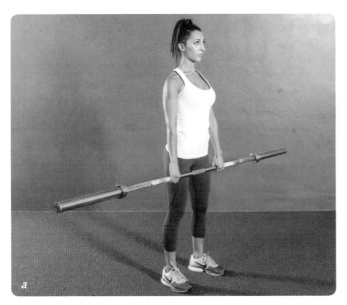
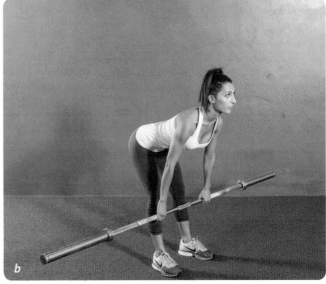

DUMBBELL STIFF-LEG DEADLIFT

This move targets the glutes and hamstrings.

Posterior Thigh and Hip Category 1

START

Stand with your feet shoulder-width apart. Grasp a pair of dumbbells and let them hang in front of you with your palms facing your body.

MOVEMENT

Keeping your knees straight, bend forward at the hips and lower the dumbbells until you feel an intense stretch in your hamstrings. Then, reverse direction, forcefully contracting your glutes as you rise up to the start position.

EXPERT TIPS

- You should bend forward only at the hips, not the low back. The action is purely hip extension; any spinal movement will place the vertebrae at risk of injury.

- There is rarely a need to stand on a box, as many people do. This is necessary only if you can touch your toes without flexing your spine—a feat very few can do.

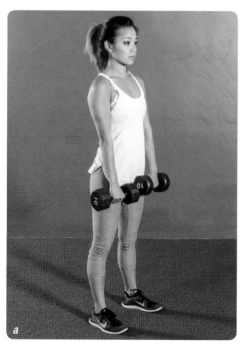 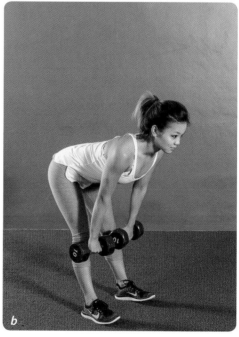

BARBELL GLUTE BRIDGE

This move targets the glutes.

Posterior Thigh and Hip Category 1

START

Lie on the floor with your legs straight and your back flat on the floor. Position a barbell over your lower legs and roll the bar over your thighs so that it is situated at the crease of your hips slightly above your pelvis. Bend your knees to a 90-degree angle, and keep your feet shoulder-width apart and your heels planted firmly on the floor.

MOVEMENT

Keeping your core braced and your spine in a neutral position, raise the barbell off the floor as high as comfortably possible by powerfully contracting your hip extensors. Squeeze your glutes for a 1-count at the top of the movement, and then return to the start position.

EXPERT TIPS

- Your knees should track directly over your toes and not cave inward.
- Focus on pushing through the entire foot while keeping the soles of your feet flat on the floor.
- Place a pad on the bar to reduce pressure on the muscles in your lower abdominal region.

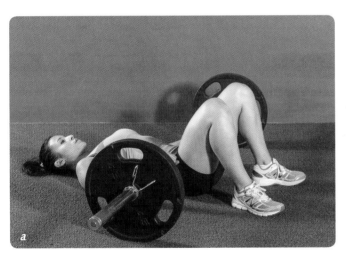
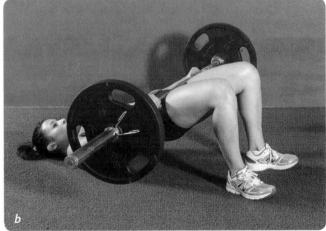

BARBELL HIP THRUST

This move targets the glutes.

Posterior Thigh and Hip Category 1

START

Sit on the floor with your legs straight, and place your upper back against a secured and padded bench (or step, box, etc.). Position a barbell over your lower legs and roll the bar over your thighs so that it is situated at the crease of your hips slightly above your pelvis. Bend your knees to a 90-degree angle, and keep your feet shoulder-width apart and planted firmly on the floor.

MOVEMENT

Keeping your core braced and your spine in a neutral position, raise the barbell off the floor by powerfully contracting your hip extensors until your torso is parallel to the floor. Squeeze your glutes for a 1-count at the top of the movement, and then return to the start position.

EXPERT TIPS

- Your knees should track directly over your toes and not cave inward.
- Focus on pushing through the entire foot while keeping the soles of your feet flat on the floor.
- Place a pad on the bar to reduce pressure on the muscles of your lower abdominal region.

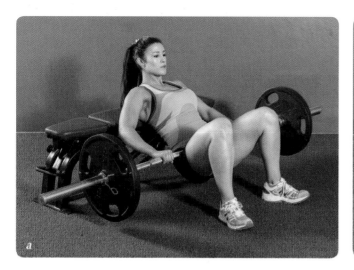
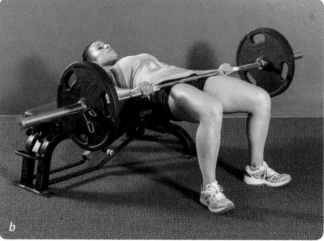

CABLE GLUTE BACK KICK

This move targets the glutes (particularly the gluteus maximus) and hamstrings.

Posterior Thigh and Hip Category 1

START

Attach a cuff to the low pulley of a cable apparatus, and then secure the cuff to your left ankle. Face the weight stack and grasp something sturdy for support.

MOVEMENT

Keeping your upper body motionless and your left leg straight, bring your left foot back as far as comfortably possible without moving your upper torso. Contract your glutes and return to the start position. After performing the desired number of reps on your left side, repeat on your right side.

EXPERT TIP

To decrease activation of the hamstrings and thereby increase activation of the glutes, bend your working knee slightly while performing the move.

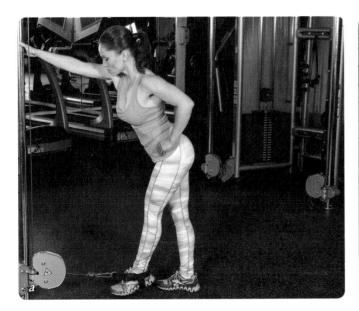
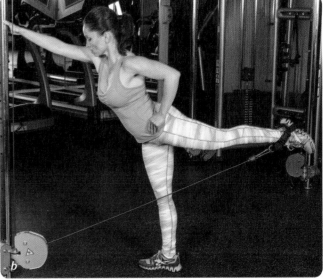

REVERSE HYPEREXTENSION

This move targets the glutes and hamstrings.

Posterior Thigh and Hip Category 1

START

Lie prone on a Roman chair, grasping the metal post underneath the roller pads. Your chest should rest on the bench pad, and your legs should hang down as far as possible without touching the floor.

MOVEMENT

Keeping your arms fixed, lift your legs until your ankles and the back of your head are in a straight line. Contract your glutes and return along the same path to the start position.

EXPERT TIPS

- Your knees should remain straight throughout the move; don't use momentum by flexing and then whipping the lower legs straight.
- Don't hyperextend the back, because this can cause lumbar injury.
- If the move becomes easy, attach leg weights to your ankles.

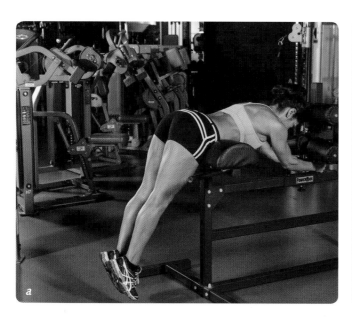 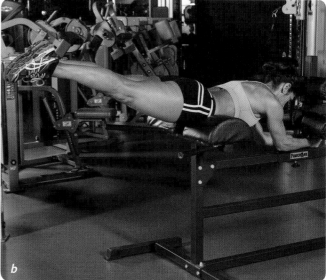

HYPEREXTENSION

This move targets the glutes and hamstrings.

Posterior Thigh and Hip Category 1

START

Lie prone on a Roman chair with your feet hooked securely underneath the roller pads and your pelvis resting on the bench pad. Cross your arms over your chest.

MOVEMENT

Keeping your lower body stable and your head up, lift your chest and shoulders until your ankles and the back of your head are in a straight line. Contract your glutes and then return along the same path to the start position.

EXPERT TIPS

- Don't move your head during the move; doing so can cause injury to your neck.
- Don't hyperextend your low back; this can cause lumbar injury.
- To increase the level of difficulty, hold a weight plate against your chest as you perform the move.

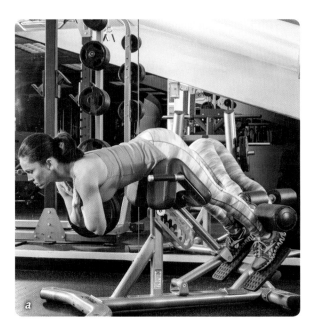
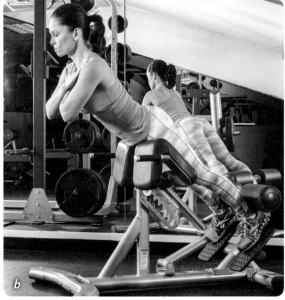

CABLE STANDING ABDUCTION

This move targets the glutes, particularly the gluteus medius and minimus, as well as the outer thigh muscles.

Posterior Thigh and Hip Category 1

START

Attach a cuff to the low pulley of a cable apparatus, and then secure the cuff to your left ankle. Position yourself so that your right side faces the weight stack, and grasp something sturdy for support. Keep your body erect and your core tight, and allow your left leg to come across your body so that it crosses over your right leg.

MOVEMENT

Keeping your upper body motionless, pull your left leg across your body and directly out to the side. Contract your glutes and then return the weight along the same path to the start position. After performing the desired number of repetitions, reverse the process and repeat on the right.

EXPERT TIPS

- To shift tension to the external rotator muscles (i.e., piriformis, gemellus, and obturators), rotate your little toe outward as you perform the move.
- Don't lean to complete the move; this introduces unwanted momentum into the lift, decreasing stimulation of the target muscle.

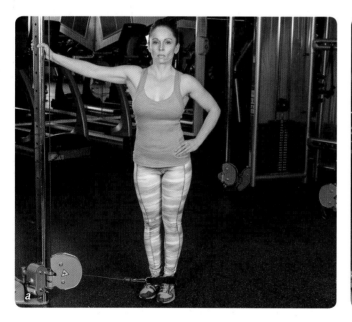 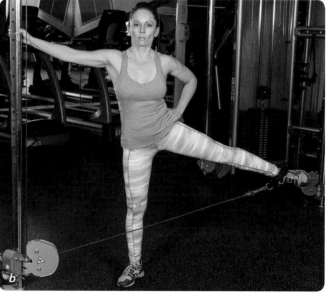

LYING LEG CURL

This move targets the hamstrings.

Posterior Thigh and Hip Category 2

START

Lie prone on a lying leg curl machine. Hook your heels underneath the roller pad. Grasp the handles (if available) or the bench pad for stability.

MOVEMENT

Keeping your thighs pressed against the bench surface, curl your feet upward, stopping just short of touching your butt, or as far as comfortably possible. Contract your hamstrings and then reverse direction, returning to the start position.

EXPERT TIP

Don't allow the moving weight stack to touch the nonmoving part of the weight stack at the start of the move. Doing so takes tension off the hamstrings.

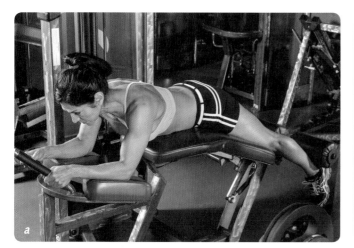
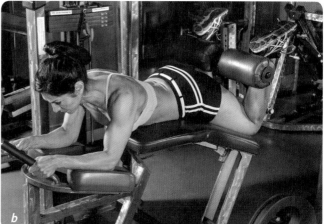

MACHINE KNEELING LEG CURL

This move targets the hamstrings.

Posterior Thigh and Hip Category 2

START

Place your left knee on the knee pad of a kneeling leg curl machine, and hook your right heel underneath the roller pad. Place your forearms on the restraint pads for support. Keep your back flat and your torso immobile throughout the move.

MOVEMENT

Curl your right foot upward, stopping just short of touching your butt, or as far as comfortably possible. Contract your right hamstring and then reverse direction, returning to the start position. After performing the desired number of repetitions, repeat the process on your left.

EXPERT TIP

Don't allow the moving weight stack to touch the nonmoving part of the weight stack at the start of the move. Doing so takes tension off the hamstrings.

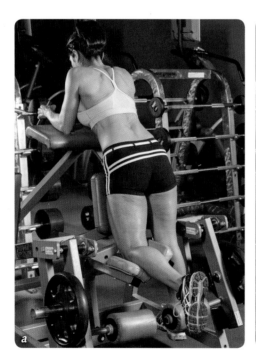
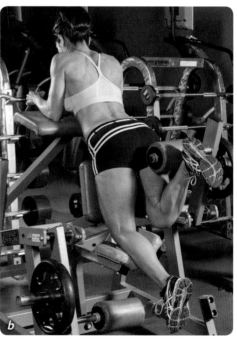

MACHINE SEATED LEG CURL

This move targets the hamstrings.

Posterior Thigh and Hip Category 2

START

Sit in a seated leg curl machine. Keep your back flat against the back rest and place your heels over the roller pads. Lower the leg restraint over your shins so that they are secure.

MOVEMENT

Press your feet downward as far as comfortably possible, contracting your hamstrings when your knees are fully bent. Then, reverse direction and return to the start position.

EXPERT TIP

Don't allow the moving weight stack to touch the nonmoving part of the weight stack at the start of the move. Doing so takes tension off the hamstrings.

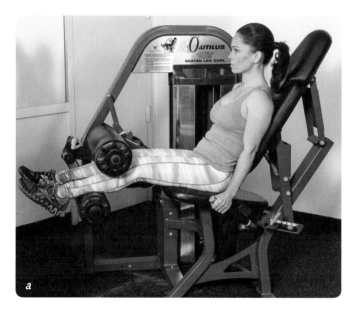 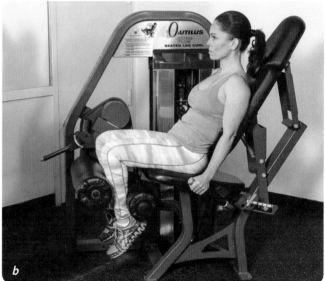

STABILITY BALL LEG CURL

This move targets the hamstrings. It's an excellent move for isolating the hamstrings without allowing the more powerful glutes to dominate.

Posterior Thigh and Hip Category 2

START

Lie supine on the floor and place your heels on top of a stability ball. Your arms should rest by your sides, and your head should be in line with your body.

MOVEMENT

Keeping your torso and thighs in a straight line, pull the ball toward you with your heels as close as possible by raising your hips off the floor. Contract your hamstrings and return along the same path to the start position.

EXPERT TIPS

- At the top of the move, the soles of your feet should be flat on the ball.
- Use a larger ball to increase range of motion.

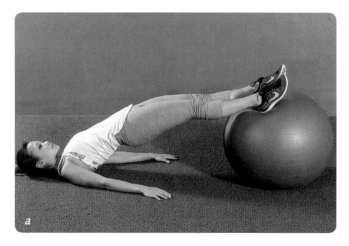
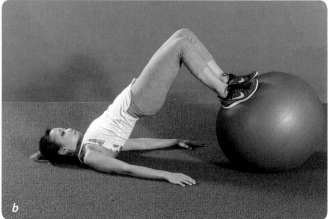

CALF EXERCISES

Exercises for the calves are divided into the following two categories (see table 4.3):

- Category 1 comprises straight-leg calf exercises.
- Category 2 comprises bent-leg calf exercises.

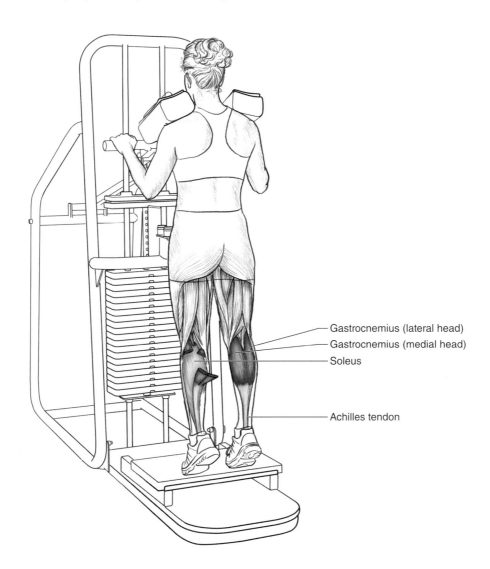

Gastrocnemius (lateral head)
Gastrocnemius (medial head)
Soleus
Achilles tendon

Table 4.3 Calf Exercises by Category

Category 1	Category 2
Toe press	Machine seated calf raise
Machine standing calf raise	Machine single-leg seated calf raise
Dumbbell standing calf raise	Seated weighted calf raise
Dumbbell single-leg standing calf raise	

TOE PRESS

This move targets the calf muscles.

Calf Category 1

START

Sit upright in a leg press unit, pressing your back firmly against the padded seat. Place the balls of your feet a comfortable distance apart on the bottom of the footplate, keeping your heels off the footplate. Straighten your legs, unlock the carriage-release bars, and drop your heels below your toes.

MOVEMENT

Keeping your knees immobile, press your toes as high up as you can until your ankles are fully extended. Contract your calves and then reverse the direction, returning to the start position.

EXPERT TIPS

- Never bounce during the stretched position of the move. Doing so can cause severe injury to the Achilles tendon.
- Turning your toes outward can place increased emphasis on the middle head of the gastrocnemius, whereas turning your toes inward can target the lateral gastrocnemius head.

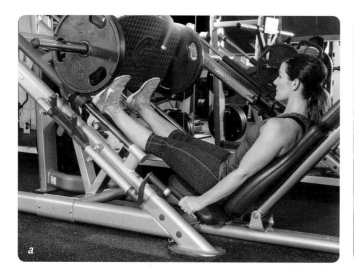
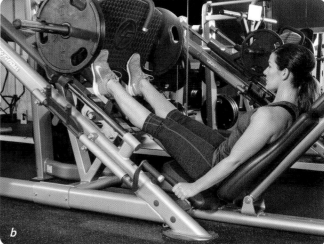

MACHINE STANDING CALF RAISE

This move targets the calves with an emphasis on the soleus muscle.

Calf Category 1

START

Place your shoulders on the restraint pads of a standing calf machine. Place the balls of your feet on the footplate, and drop your heels below your toes.

MOVEMENT

Rise as high as you can onto your toes until your ankles are fully extended. Contract your calves and then reverse direction, returning to the start position.

EXPERT TIPS

- Never bounce at the stretched position of the move. Doing so can cause severe injury to the Achilles tendon.
- Turning your toes outward can place increased emphasis on the middle head of the gastrocnemius, whereas turning your toes inward can target the lateral gastrocnemius head.

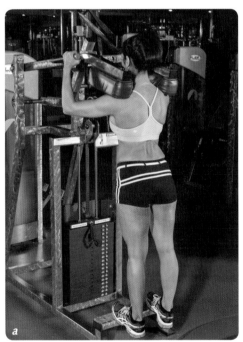 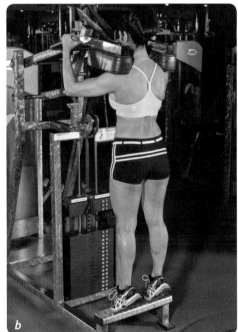

DUMBBELL STANDING CALF RAISE

This move targets the calves.

Calf Category 1

START

Stand on a step (such as a block of wood or staircase) and allow your heels to drop below your toes. Hold on to a stationary object with one hand, and hold a dumbbell in the other hand.

MOVEMENT

Rise as high as you can onto your toes until your calves are fully extended. Contract your calves and then reverse direction, returning to the start position.

EXPERT TIP

Never bounce at the stretched position of the move. Doing so can cause severe injury to the Achilles tendon.

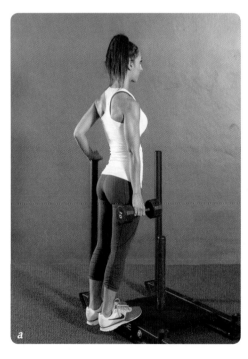 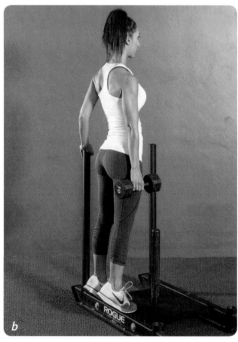

DUMBBELL SINGLE-LEG STANDING CALF RAISE

This move targets the calves.

Calf Category 1

START

Stand on a step (such as a block of wood or staircase), bring your left leg behind your body, and allow your right heel to drop below your toes. Hold on to a stationary object with one hand, and hold a dumbbell in the other hand.

MOVEMENT

Rise as high as you can onto your right toes until your calf muscles are fully extended. Contract your calf muscles and then reverse direction, returning to the start position. After performing the desired number of reps, repeat the process on your left side.

EXPERT TIP

Never bounce at the stretched position of the move. Doing so can cause severe injury to the Achilles tendon.

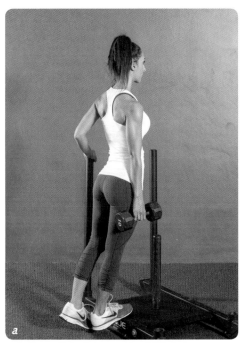 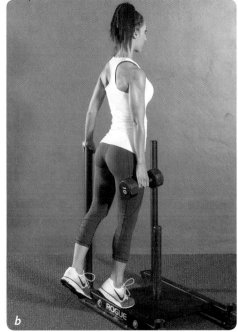

MACHINE SEATED CALF RAISE

This move targets the calves with an emphasis on the soleus muscle.

Calf Category 2

START

Sit in a seated calf machine and place the restraint pads tightly across your thighs. Place the balls of your feet on the footplate, and drop your heels as far below your toes as possible.

MOVEMENT

Rise as high as you can onto your toes until your ankles are fully extended. Contract your calves and then reverse direction, returning to the start position.

EXPERT TIPS

- Never bounce at the stretched position of the move. Doing so can cause severe injury to the Achilles tendon.
- Because the gastrocnemius muscle is not very active in this exercise, it is best to keep your toes pointed straight ahead.

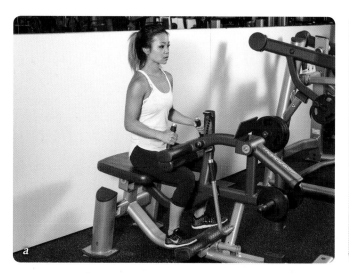 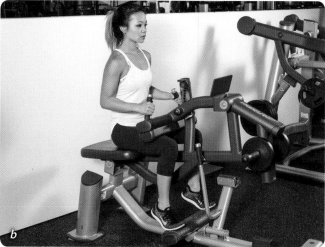

MACHINE SINGLE-LEG SEATED CALF RAISE

This move targets the calves with an emphasis on the soleus muscle.

Calf Category 2

START

Sit in a seated calf machine and place the restraint pads tightly across your thighs. Place the ball of your right foot on the footplate, and drop your right heel as far below your toes as possible. Bend your left knee and let it drop down so that it does not assist in the move.

MOVEMENT

Rise as high as you can onto your toes until your ankle is fully extended. Contract your right calf muscles and then reverse direction, returning to the start position. After performing the desired number of repetitions, repeat on your left side.

EXPERT TIPS

- Never bounce at the stretched position of the move. Doing so can cause severe injury to the Achilles tendon.
- Because the gastrocnemius muscle is not very active in this exercise, it is best to keep your toes pointed straight ahead.

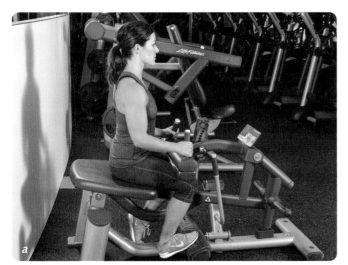
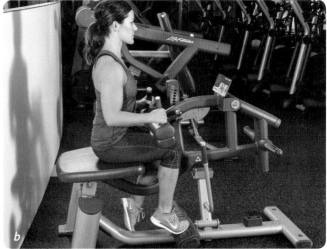

SEATED WEIGHTED CALF RAISE

This move targets the calves with an emphasis on the soleus muscle.

Calf Category 2

START

Sit at the edge of a flat bench with the balls of your feet on a block of wood or step. Place a dumbbell or weighted plate on your thighs, and hold it in place while dropping your heels as far below your toes as possible.

MOVEMENT

Rise as high as you can onto your toes until your calves are fully extended. Contract your calves and then reverse direction, returning to the start position.

EXPERT TIPS

- Never bounce at the stretched position of the move. Doing so can cause severe injury to the Achilles tendon.
- Keep your toes pointed straight ahead. Significant outward or inward rotation places the knee in a position of poor tracking and can lead to injury (and contrary to popular belief, will not work the calf muscles any differently).
- For added comfort, place a folded towel on your thighs underneath the weights.

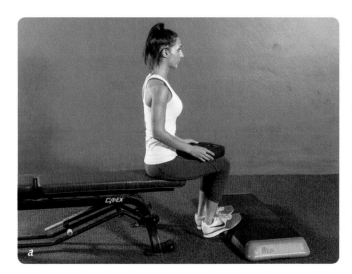
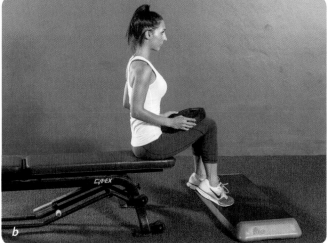

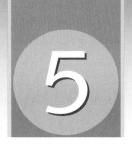

Exercises for the Torso

This chapter describes and illustrates exercises for the muscles of the torso. Read the descriptions carefully, and scrutinize the photos to ensure proper form. I have provided expert tips for each of these movements to optimize your training performance. Remember that exercises are merely tools, or a means to an end—in this case, for enhancing muscular development. If an exercise does not feel right to you, simply substitute it for a comparable move.

BACK EXERCISES

Exercises for the back are divided into the following three categories (see table 5.1):

- Category 1 comprises exercises involving multijoint pull-ups and pull-downs.
- Category 2 comprises exercises involving multijoint rowing movements.
- Category 3 comprises exercises involving single-joint movements targeting the back musculature.

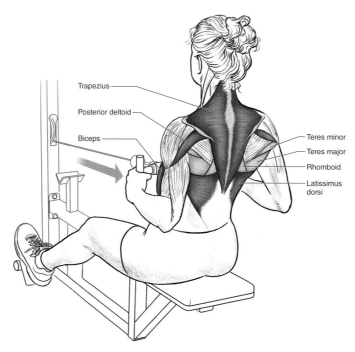

Table 5.1 Back Exercises by Category

Category 1	Category 2	Category 3
Chin-up	Dumbbell single-arm row	Dumbbell pullover
Pull-up	T-bar row	Cable straight-arm pull-down
Lat pull-down	Barbell reverse bent row	
Neutral-grip lat pull-down	Cable seated row	
Reverse-grip lat pull-down	Cable wide-grip seated row	
Cross cable pull-down	Machine seated row	
	Machine wide-grip seated row	
	Cable single-arm standing low row	
	Inverted row	

CHIN-UP

This move targets the back muscles with secondary emphasis on the biceps. It's a bit easier to perform than the pull-up.

Back Category 1

START

Grasp a chinning bar with an underhand, shoulder-width grip (palms facing your body). Straighten your arms, bend your knees, and cross one foot over the other.

MOVEMENT

Keeping your upper body stable, pull your body up until your chin reaches the bar. Contract your lats and then return along the same path to the start position.

EXPERT TIPS

- Don't allow your body to swing; this introduces unwanted momentum into the movement.
- This can be a very difficult move to execute, especially for those who carry more weight in the lower body. If you can't reach your target rep range, place your feet on a chair and push up to bring your chin to the bar; then lift your feet from the chair and lower yourself. Performing slow negatives in this fashion will help you develop strength in the move.
- Alternatively, you can use an assisted device such as the Gravitron if your gym has one.

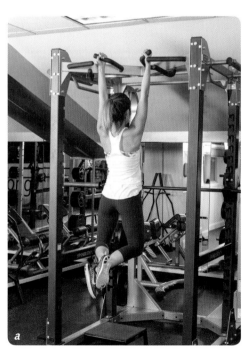
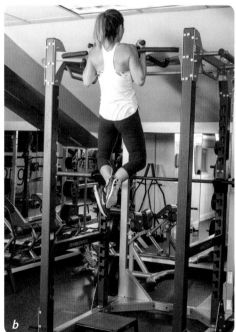

PULL-UP

This move targets the back muscles.

Back Category 1

START

Grasp a chinning bar with an overhand, shoulder-width grip (palms facing away from your body). Straighten your arms, bend your knees, and cross one foot over the other.

MOVEMENT

Keeping your upper body stable, pull your body up until your chin reaches the bar. Contract your lats and then return along the same path to the start position.

EXPERT TIPS

- Don't allow your body to swing; this introduces momentum into the movement, reducing tension to the target muscles.
- This can be a very difficult move to execute, especially for those who carry more weight in the lower body. If you can't reach your target rep range, place your feet on a chair and push up to bring your chin to the bar; then lift your feet from the chair and lower yourself. Performing slow negatives in this fashion will help you develop strength in the move.
- Alternatively, you can use an assisted device such as the Gravitron if your gym has one.

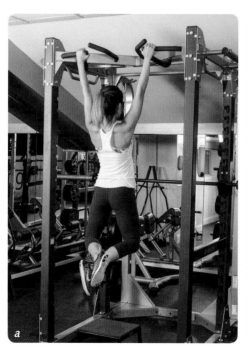 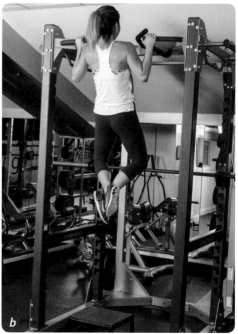

LAT PULL-DOWN

This move targets the back muscles, particularly the lats.

Back Category 1

START

Grasp a straight bar attached to the lat pull-down machine. With your hands shoulder-width apart and palms turned forward, secure your knees under the restraint pad and fully straighten your arms so that you feel a complete stretch in your lats. Maintain a slight backward tilt and keep your low back arched throughout the move.

MOVEMENT

Pull the bar down to your upper chest. Squeeze your shoulder blades together and then reverse direction, returning to the start position.

EXPERT TIPS

- Don't lean back too far. Doing so turns the move into a row rather than a pull-down.
- Don't swing your body as your perform the move. This introduces excessive momentum into the lift, reducing tension on the target musculature.

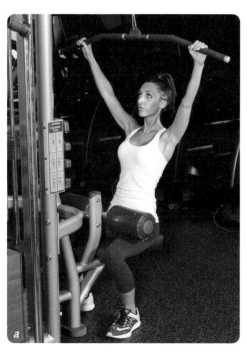 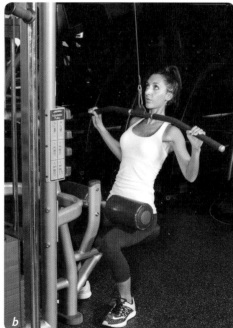

NEUTRAL-GRIP LAT PULL-DOWN

This move targets the back muscles.

Back Category 1

START

Grasp a V-bar attached to a lat pull-down machine. Secure your knees under the restraint pad, and fully straighten your arms so that you feel a complete stretch in your lats. Maintain a slight backward tilt to your body and keep your low back arched throughout the move.

MOVEMENT

Pull the bar down to your upper chest. Squeeze your shoulder blades together and then reverse direction, returning to the start position.

EXPERT TIPS

- Don't lean back too far. Doing so turns the move into a row rather than a pull-down.
- Don't swing your body as your perform the move. This introduces unwanted momentum into the lift, reducing tension on the target musculature.

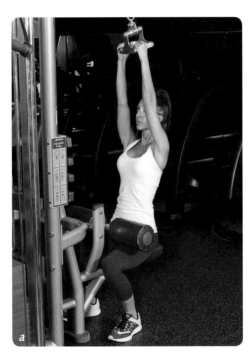 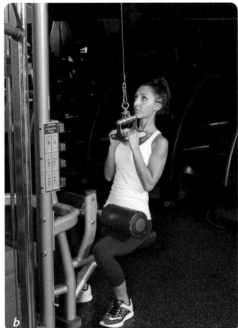

REVERSE-GRIP LAT PULL-DOWN

This move targets the back muscles.

Back Category 1

START

Grasp a lat pull-down bar with your hands shoulder-width apart and your palms turned toward you. Secure your knees under the restraint pad, and fully straighten your arms so that you feel a complete stretch in your lats. Maintain a slight backward tilt to your body and keep your low back arched throughout the move.

MOVEMENT

Pull the bar to your upper chest. Squeeze your shoulder blades together and then reverse direction, returning to the start position.

EXPERT TIPS

- Don't lean back too far. Doing so turns the move into a row rather than a pull-down.
- Don't swing your body as your perform the move. This introduces excessive momentum into the lift, reducing tension on the target musculature.

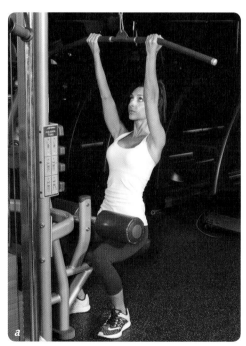 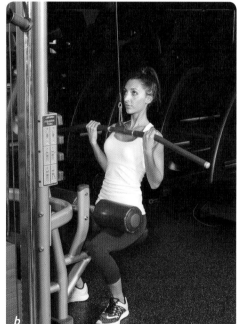

CROSS CABLE PULL-DOWN

This move targets the back muscles, particularly the lats.

Back Category 1

START

Grasp the loop handles of a high pulley attached to a cable apparatus. Kneel on the floor, facing away from the apparatus, and allow your arms to extend fully so that you feel a stretch in your lat muscles. Your palms should face away from your body, and your low back should be slightly arched.

MOVEMENT

Keeping your body stable, pull the handles down and toward your sides. Contract your lats and then reverse direction, returning to the start position.

EXPERT TIP

Don't allow your elbows to move forward during the move; this changes the plane of the exercise and thus alters muscle recruitment.

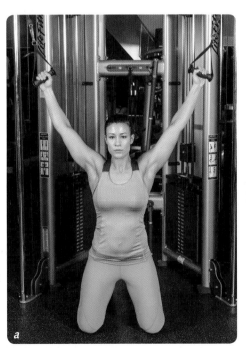
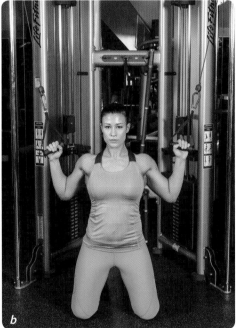

DUMBBELL SINGLE-ARM ROW

This move targets the back muscles and is especially effective for developing the inner back musculature.

Back Category 2

START

Place your left hand and left knee on a flat bench with your right foot planted firmly on the floor. Grasp a dumbbell in your right hand with your palm facing the bench, and let it hang by your side.

MOVEMENT

Keeping your elbow close to your body, pull the dumbbell up until it almost touches your side. Feel a contraction in your upper back and then reverse direction, returning to the start position. Repeat with your left arm after performing the desired number of reps on your right.

EXPERT TIPS

- Keep your back slightly arched and your torso parallel to the floor throughout the movement.
- Keep your chin up at all times; this helps prevent rounding of the spine.

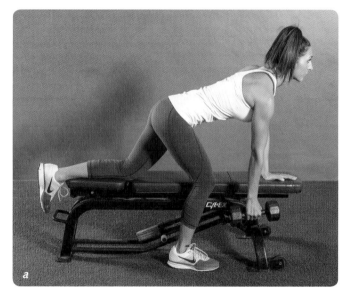
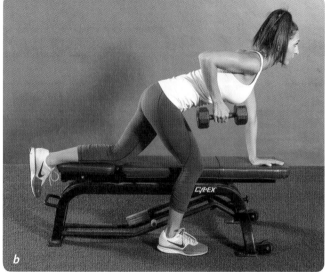

T-BAR ROW

This move targets the back muscles.

Back Category 2

START

Stand in a T-bar unit with the bar between your legs and your feet shoulder-width apart, and grasp the upper portion of the bar with both hands (one hand above the other). Bend forward slightly at the hips, keep your core tight, and allow the bar to hang down in front of your body.

MOVEMENT

Keeping your elbows close to your sides, pull the bar up into your midsection as high as possible. Contract the muscles in your upper back and then reverse direction, returning to the start position.

EXPERT TIPS

- If you don't have access to a T-bar unit, wrap a towel around one end of a bar and place it in the corner of the room (the towel will help prevent damage to the wall) and perform as described.

- Maintaining a slight hyperextension of the low back is extremely important. Any spinal bend can result in lumbar injury.

- Keep your head up at all times; this helps to prevent rounding of the spine.

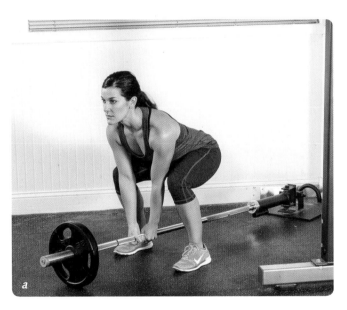
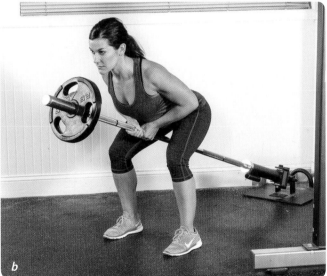

BARBELL REVERSE BENT ROW

This move targets the back muscles.

Back Category 2

START

Grasp a barbell with a shoulder-width reverse grip (palms facing away from your body). Stand with your upper body angled forward, your knees bent, and your low back slightly arched. Allow your arms to hang straight down from your shoulders.

MOVEMENT

Keeping your elbows close to your sides, pull the bar up into your midsection as high as possible. Contract the muscles in your upper back and then reverse direction, returning to the start position.

EXPERT TIPS

- Maintaining a slight hyperextension of the low back is extremely important. Any spinal bend can result in lumbar injury.
- Keep your head up at all times; this helps to prevent rounding of the spine.

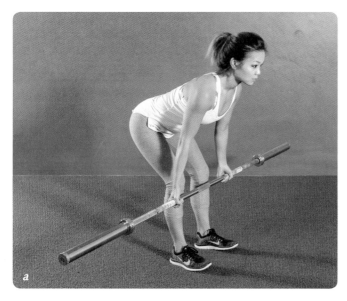
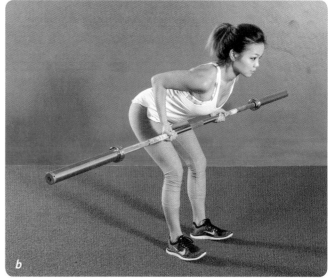

CABLE SEATED ROW

This move targets the back muscles, particularly the inner musculature of the rhomboids and the middle traps.

Back Category 2

START

Grasp a V-bar attached to a seated cable apparatus with your palms facing each other. Sit upright on the padded seat and place your feet against the footrests. Fully straighten your arms so that you feel a complete stretch in your lats. Make sure your posture is erect, with a slight arch in your low back.

MOVEMENT

Maintaining a slight bend in your knees, pull the handles in toward your lower abdomen, keeping your elbows close to your sides and your low back tight. As the handles touch your body, squeeze your shoulder blades together and then reverse the direction, returning to the start position.

EXPERT TIPS

- Don't lean forward on the return. This injects unwanted momentum into the move on the concentric action, reducing tension to the target muscles.
- Never round your spine; this places the discs in a precarious position and can lead to serious injury.

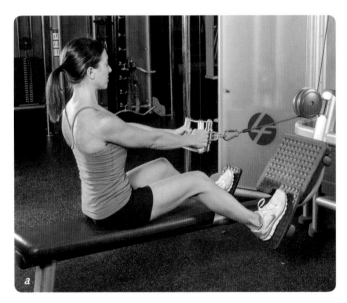 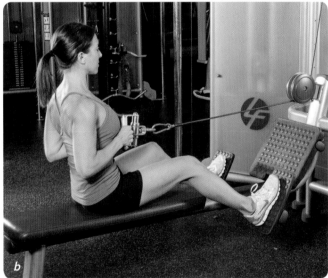

CABLE WIDE-GRIP SEATED ROW

This move targets the back muscles as well as the posterior deltoids.

Back Category 2

START

Grasp the handles of a long bar attached to a seated cable apparatus with a grip that is wider than shoulder width. Sit upright on the padded seat and place your feet against the footrests. Fully straighten your arms so that you feel a complete stretch in your lats. Make sure your posture is erect, with a slight arch in your low back.

MOVEMENT

Maintaining a slight bend in your knees, pull the bar in toward your lower abdomen, keeping your elbows close to your sides and your low back tight. As the bar touches your body, squeeze your shoulder blades together and then reverse the direction, returning to the start position.

EXPERT TIPS

- Don't lean forward on the return. This injects momentum into the move on the concentric action, reducing tension to the target muscles.
- Never round your spine; this places the discs in a precarious position and can lead to serious injury.

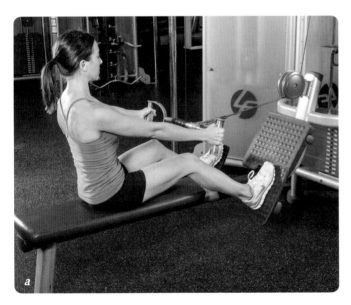 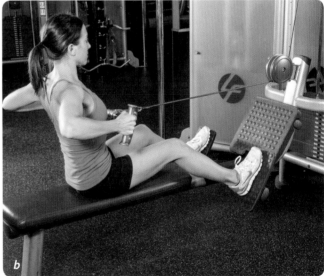

MACHINE SEATED ROW

This move targets the back muscles, particularly the inner musculature of the rhomboids and the middle traps.

Back Category 2

START

Sit with the front of your body facing the pad of a seated row unit. Press your chest against the pad, if possible, and grasp the machine handles with a neutral grip (palms facing each other). Adjust the seat height so that when you grasp the handles, your arms are fully extended and you feel a stretch in your lats.

MOVEMENT

Keeping your elbows close to your sides and your low back slightly arched, pull the handles back as far as possible without discomfort. Squeeze your shoulder blades together and then reverse the direction, returning to the start position.

EXPERT TIP

Don't swing your body forward at the beginning of the move. I see this common mistake far too often. It serves only to overstress the low back muscles and inject unwanted momentum into the move.

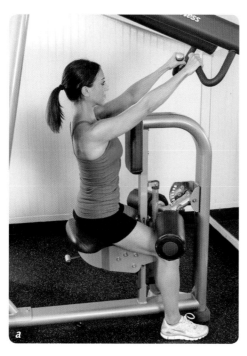
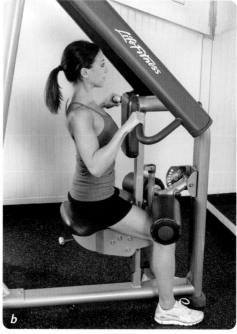

MACHINE WIDE-GRIP SEATED ROW

This move targets the back muscles as well as the posterior deltoids.

Back Category 2

START

Sit with the front of your body facing the pad of a seated row unit. Press your chest against the pad, and grasp the machine handles with a grip that is wider than shoulder width. Adjust the seat height so that when you grasp the handles, your arms are fully extended and you feel a stretch in your lats.

MOVEMENT

Keeping your elbows flared and your low back slightly arched, pull the handles back as far as possible without discomfort. Squeeze your shoulder blades together and then reverse the direction, returning to the start position.

EXPERT TIP

Don't swing your body forward at the beginning of the move. I see this common mistake far too often. It serves only to overstress the low back muscles and inject unwanted momentum into the move.

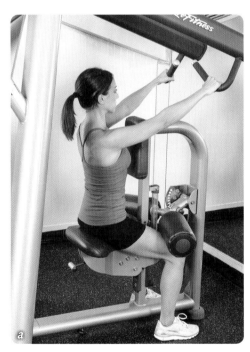 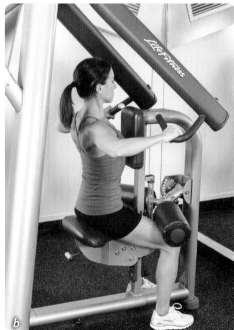

CABLE SINGLE-ARM STANDING LOW ROW

This move targets the back muscles, particularly the rhomboids and middle traps.

Back Category 2

START

Grasp the loop handle of a low pulley attached to a cable apparatus with your left hand, using a neutral grip (palm facing in). Step back from the machine and straighten your left arm so that you feel a stretch in your left lat. Keep your left leg back and bend your right leg so that your weight is forward. Place your right hand on your right knee for balance (or, if desired, hold on to the machine with your right hand).

MOVEMENT

Pull the loop handle toward your left side, keeping your elbow close to your body. Contract your left lat and then reverse direction, returning to the start position. Repeat with your right arm after performing the desired number of reps on your left.

EXPERT TIPS

- Never round your spine; this places the discs in a precarious position and can lead to serious injury.
- Avoid twisting your body as you pull the weight up; this not only results in unwanted momentum, but also can lead to spinal injury.

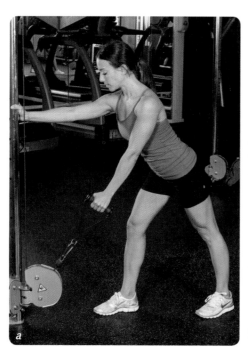 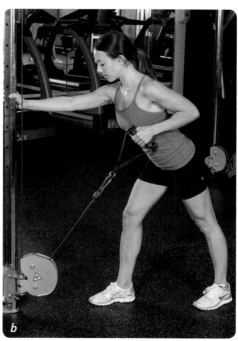

INVERTED ROW

This move targets the back musculature.

Back Category 2

START

Position yourself in a Smith machine with the bar adjusted to approximately waist height. Grasp the bar with a grip slightly wider than shoulder width, palms facing your body. Descend so that you are hanging underneath the bar with your torso and lower body forming a straight line at a 60-degree angle. Your feet should be flat on the floor, and your arms should be fully extended.

MOVEMENT

Keeping your body straight and spine neutral, pull your chest up toward the bar. Squeeze your shoulder blades together at the top of the movement, and then return to the start position.

EXPERT TIPS

- To make the move easier, decrease the angle of your body at the start position; to make the move harder, increase the starting angle.
- To decrease biceps involvement, use an overhand grip on the bar.
- You can perform this move with a suspension trainer, which adds a level of instability that activates the core to a greater degree.

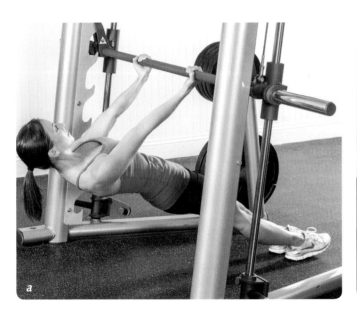 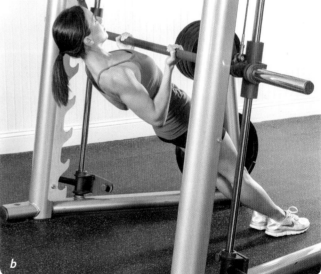

DUMBBELL PULLOVER

This move targets the lats and middle part of the chest.

Back Category 3

START

Lie supine (faceup) on a flat bench with your feet firmly planted on the floor. Grasp a dumbbell with both hands and raise it directly over your face.

MOVEMENT

Keeping your elbows slightly bent, lower the dumbbell behind your head as far as comfortably possible. When you feel a complete stretch in your lats, forcefully reverse direction and return to the start position.

EXPERT TIPS

- Stretch only to the point of comfort; overstretching can lead to shoulder injury.
- Your elbows should maintain a slight bend throughout the movement. Do not straighten as you lift, because this will increase triceps activation at the expense of your target muscles.

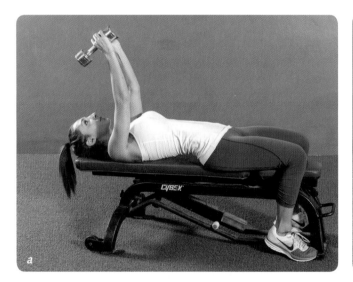
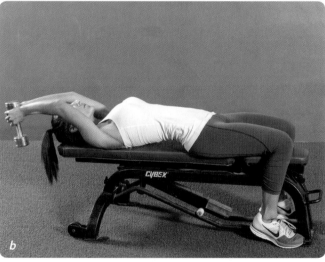

CABLE STRAIGHT-ARM PULL-DOWN

This move targets the back muscles, particularly the lats.

Back Category 3

START

Take an overhand, shoulder-width grip on a straight bar attached to a high pulley. Slightly bend your elbows and bring the bar to shoulder level. Your feet should be approximately shoulder-width apart, your knees should be slightly bent, and your core should be tight.

MOVEMENT

Keeping a slight forward tilt to your upper body, pull the bar down in a semicircle until it touches your upper thighs. Contract your back muscles and then reverse the direction, returning to the start position.

EXPERT TIP

This move can be performed with a variety of handle attachments, such as a rope, curved bar, and loop handles.

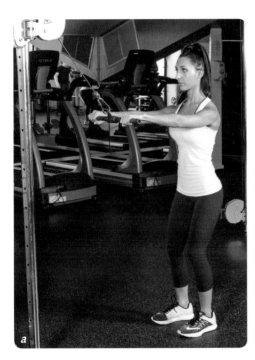 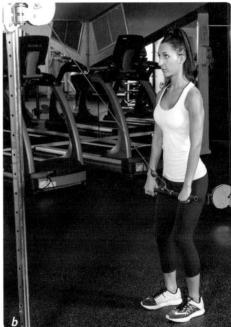

CHEST EXERCISES

Exercises for the chest are divided into the following four categories (see table 5.2):

- Category 1 comprises multijoint exercises targeting the upper-chest musculature.
- Category 2 comprises multijoint exercises targeting the midchest musculature.
- Category 3 comprises single-joint exercises targeting the upper-chest musculature.
- Category 4 comprises single-joint exercises targeting the midchest musculature.

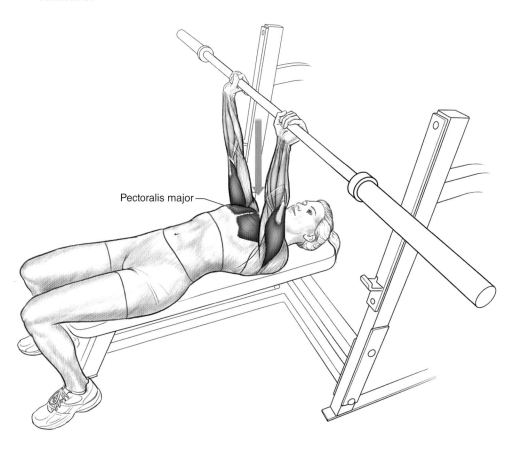

Pectoralis major

Table 5.2 Chest Exercises by Category

Category 1	Category 2	Category 3	Category 4
Dumbbell incline press	Dumbbell decline press	Dumbbell incline fly	Flat dumbbell fly
Barbell incline press	Dumbbell chest press	Low cable fly	Mid cable fly
Machine incline press	Barbell decline press		Pec deck fly
	Barbell chest press		
	Machine chest press		

DUMBBELL INCLINE PRESS

This move targets the pectorals, with an emphasis on the upper aspect of the chest. The triceps and front delts also receive significant activation.

Chest Category 1

START

Lie faceup on an incline bench set at approximately 30 to 40 degrees with your feet planted firmly on the floor. Grasp two dumbbells and, with your palms facing away from your body, bring them to shoulder level so that they rest just above your armpits.

MOVEMENT

Simultaneously press both dumbbells directly over your chest, moving them in toward each other on the ascent. At the end of the movement, the sides of the dumbbells should gently touch, and the weights should be over the upper portion of your chest. Feel a contraction in your chest muscles and then reverse direction, returning to the start position.

EXPERT TIPS

- Keep your elbows flared throughout the move to maintain maximal activation of the pecs.
- As you press the weight, think of moving them in an inverted-V pattern to increase range of motion.
- Your body should remain on the bench throughout the movement and remain stable at all times.
- To maintain continuous muscular tension, do not lock your elbows at the end of the move.

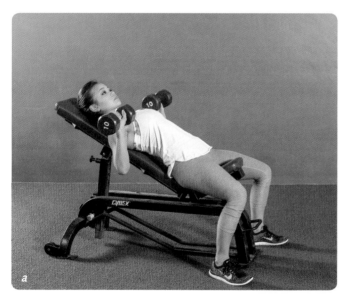
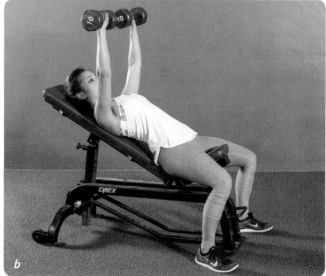

BARBELL INCLINE PRESS

This move targets the pectorals, with an emphasis on the upper aspect of the chest. The triceps and front delts also receive significant work.

Chest Category 1

START

Lie faceup on an incline bench set at approximately 30 to 40 degrees with your feet planted firmly on the floor. Grasp a barbell with a shoulder-width grip and bring it down to the upper aspect of your chest.

MOVEMENT

Press the bar directly over your upper chest, moving it in a straight line. At the end of the movement, the bar should be over the upper portion of your chest. Contract your chest muscles and then return the bar along the same path to the start position.

EXPERT TIPS

- Keep your elbows flared throughout the move.
- Your body should remain on the bench throughout the movement and remain stable at all times.
- To maintain continuous muscular tension, do not lock your elbows at the end of the move.

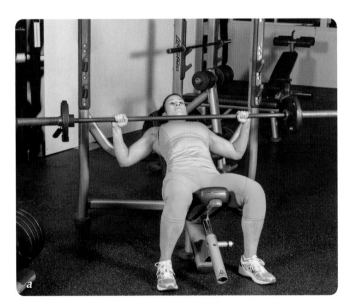
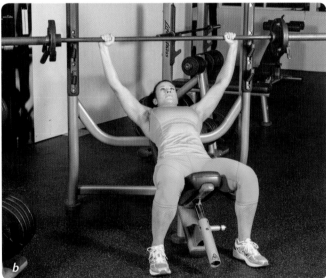

MACHINE INCLINE PRESS

This move targets the pectorals, particularly the upper portion. Secondary emphasis is on the shoulders and the triceps.

Chest Category 1

START

Sit in an incline press unit set at approximately 30 to 40 degrees, aligning your upper chest with the handles on the machine. Grasp the handles with a shoulder-width grip. Keep your palms facing away from your body and your elbows flared.

MOVEMENT

Keeping your back against the support pad, press the handles forward, stopping just before you fully lock your elbows. Feel a contraction in your chest muscles at the end of the movement and then reverse the direction, returning to the start position.

EXPERT TIPS

- Some units have the capacity to move the grade of the bench to 30 or 40 degrees to optimally target the upper chest in the incline press. However, the grade varies depending on the machine. The most important thing to remember is that the action should move in line with the upper portion of your chest. A muscle always contracts maximally when the action is carried out in line with its fibers.

- Keep your elbows flared as you lift; allowing them to move forward changes the scope of the exercise.

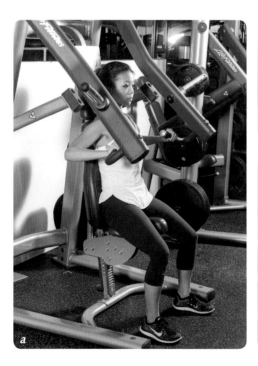
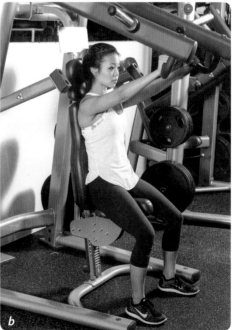

DUMBBELL DECLINE PRESS

This move targets the pectorals, with an emphasis on the lower aspect of the muscle. The triceps also receive significant activation.

Chest Category 2

START

Lie faceup on a decline bench set at approximately 30 to 40 degrees with your feet planted firmly on the floor or locked under the foot pads. Grasp two dumbbells and, with your palms facing away from your body, bring them to shoulder level so that they rest just above your armpits.

MOVEMENT

Simultaneously press both dumbbells directly over your chest, moving them in toward each other on the ascent. At the end of the movement, the sides of the dumbbells should gently touch, and the weights should be over the lower portion of your chest. Feel a contraction in your chest muscles and then reverse direction, returning to the start position.

EXPERT TIPS

- Keep your elbows flared throughout the move to maintain maximal activation of the pecs.
- As you press the dumbbells, think of moving them in an inverted-V pattern to increase range of motion.
- Your body should remain on the bench throughout the movement and remain stable at all times.
- To maintain continuous muscular tension, do not lock your elbows at the end of the move.

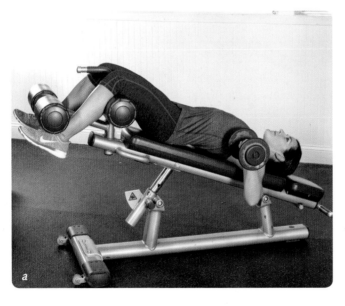
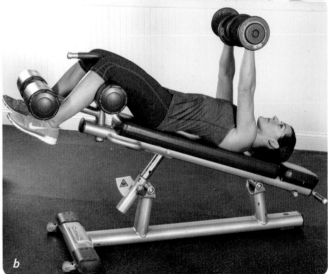

DUMBBELL CHEST PRESS

This move targets the pectorals, with an emphasis on the middle part of the chest.

Chest Category 2

START

Lie faceup on a flat bench with your feet planted firmly on the floor. Grasp two dumbbells and, with your palms facing away from your body, bring them to shoulder level so that they rest just above your armpits.

MOVEMENT

Simultaneously press both dumbbells directly over your chest, moving them in toward each other on the ascent. At the end of the movement, the sides of the dumbbells should gently touch, and the weights should be over the middle portion of your chest. Feel a contraction in your chest muscles and then reverse direction, returning to the start position.

EXPERT TIPS

- Keep your elbows flared throughout the move to maintain maximal activation of the pecs.
- As you press the dumbbells, think of moving them in an inverted-V pattern to increase range of motion.
- Your body should remain on the bench throughout the movement and remain stable at all times.
- To maintain continuous muscular tension, do not lock your elbows at the end of the move.

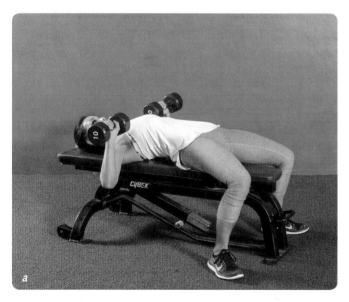
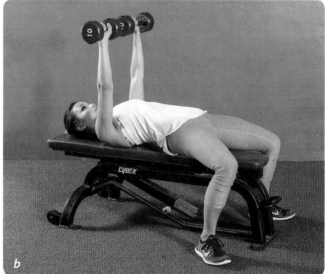

BARBELL DECLINE PRESS

This move targets the pectorals, with an emphasis on the lower aspect of the chest. The triceps and front delts also receive significant work.

Chest Category 2

START

Lie faceup on a decline bench set at approximately 30 to 40 degrees with your feet planted firmly on the floor or locked under the foot pads. Grasp a barbell with a shoulder-width grip and bring it down to the middle of your chest.

MOVEMENT

Press the bar directly over your chest, moving it in a straight line. At the end of the movement, the bar should be over the lower portion of your chest. Contract your chest muscles and then return the bar along the same path to the start position.

EXPERT TIPS

- Keep your elbows flared throughout the move.
- Your body should remain on the bench throughout the movement and remain stable at all times.
- To maintain continuous muscular tension, do not lock your elbows at the finish of the move.

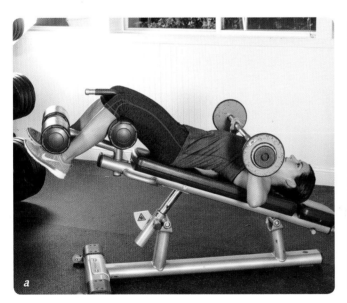 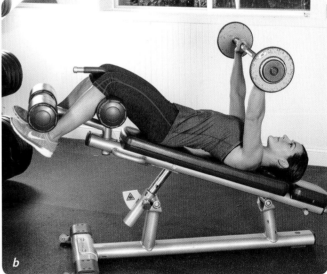

BARBELL CHEST PRESS

This move targets the pectorals, with an emphasis on the middle part of the chest. The triceps and front delts also receive significant work.

Chest Category 2

START

Lie faceup on a flat bench with your feet planted firmly on the floor. Grasp a barbell with a shoulder-width grip and bring it down to the middle of your chest.

MOVEMENT

Press the bar directly over your chest, moving it in a straight line. At the end of the movement, the bar should be over the middle portion of your chest. Contract your chest muscles and then return the bar along the same path to the start position.

EXPERT TIPS

- Keep your elbows flared throughout the move.
- Your body should remain on the bench throughout the movement and remain stable at all times.
- To maintain continuous muscular tension, do not lock your elbows at the end of the move.

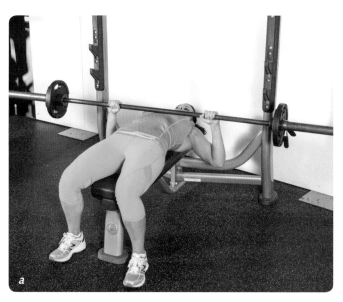
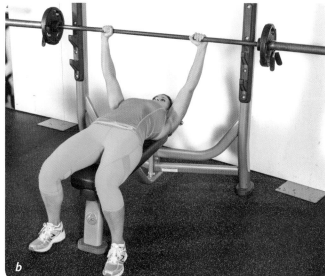

MACHINE CHEST PRESS

Chest Category 2

START

Sit in a chest press machine, aligning your upper chest with the handles on the machine. Grasp the handles with a shoulder-width grip, keeping your palms facing away from your body.

MOVEMENT

Press the handles forward, stopping just before you fully lock out your elbows. Feel a contraction in your chest muscles at the end of the movement, and then reverse direction, returning to the start position.

EXPERT TIP

Keep your elbows flared as you lift so they remain approximately parallel to the floor. Allowing them to move forward changes the plane of the exercise and thus muscle recruitment.

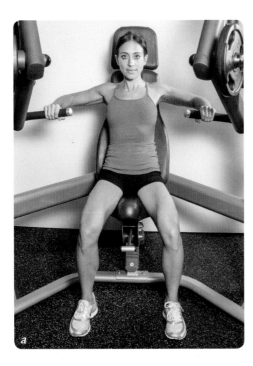 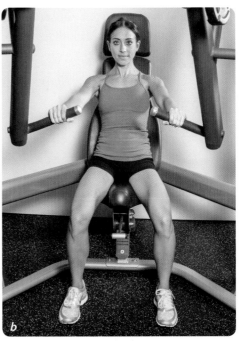

DUMBBELL INCLINE FLY

This move targets the pectorals, primarily the upper fibers. It provides better isolation for the chest muscles than an incline press does.

Chest Category 3

START

Lie supine on an incline bench set at approximately 30 to 40 degrees, and plant your feet firmly on the floor, if possible. Grasp two dumbbells and bring them out to your sides, maintaining a slight bend to your elbows throughout the move. Your palms should be facing in and toward the ceiling, and your upper arms should be roughly parallel to the level of the bench.

MOVEMENT

Raise the weights in a circular motion, gently touching them together at the top of the move. At the end of the movement, the dumbbells should be over the upper portion of your chest. Contract your chest muscles and then return the weights along the same path to the start position.

EXPERT TIPS

- Keep your arms rigidly rounded throughout the move; do not straighten your elbows.
- As you lift the weights, think of hugging a beach ball.
- Your body should remain on the bench throughout the movement and remain stable at all times.
- Avoid overstretching in the start position because doing so can cause injury.

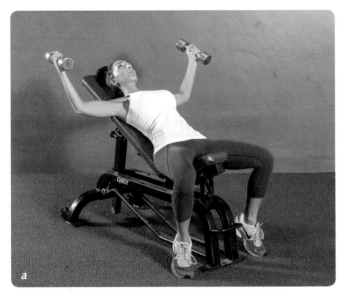
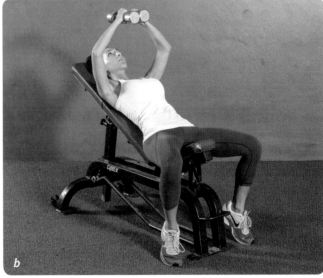

LOW CABLE FLY

This move targets the chest muscles, particularly the upper portion.

Chest Category 3

START

Grasp the handles of a pulley attached to a cable apparatus, and adjust the height so that they are slightly above floor level. Face away from the apparatus. Stand with your feet about shoulder-width apart, with one foot in front of the other, your torso bent slightly forward at the waist, and your arms slightly bent and held out to the sides so they are lower than parallel to the floor.

MOVEMENT

Keeping your upper body motionless and your core muscles tight, pull both handles up and across your body, creating a semicircular movement. Bring your hands together at the level of your chest, and squeeze your chest muscles so that you feel a contraction in the cleavage area. Then, reverse the direction, allowing your hands to return along the same path to the start position.

EXPERT TIP

Your elbows should remain slightly bent and fixed throughout the move; don't flex or extend them at any time. This error effectively makes the exercise a pressing movement rather than a fly.

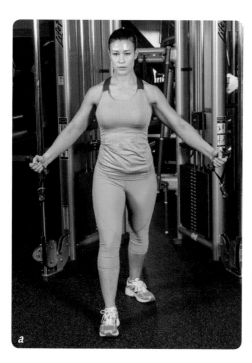
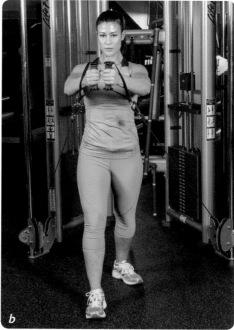

FLAT DUMBBELL FLY

This move targets the pectorals, primarily the middle fibers. It provides better isolation for the chest muscles than the flat press does.

Chest Category 4

START

Lie supine on a flat bench and plant your feet firmly on the floor. Grasp two dumbbells and bring them out to your sides, maintaining a slight bend to your elbows throughout the move. Your palms should be facing in and toward the ceiling, and your upper arms should be roughly parallel to the level of the bench.

MOVEMENT

Raise the weights in a semicircular motion, gently touching them together at the top of the move. At the end of the movement, the dumbbells should be over the upper portion of your chest. Contract your chest muscles and then return the weights along the same path to the start position.

EXPERT TIPS

- Keep your arms rigidly rounded throughout the move; do not straighten your elbows.
- As you lift the weights, think of hugging a beach ball.
- Your body should remain on the bench throughout the movement and remain stable at all times.
- Avoid overstretching in the start position because doing so can cause injury.

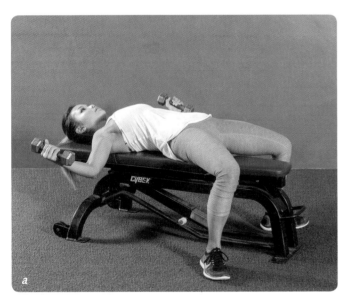

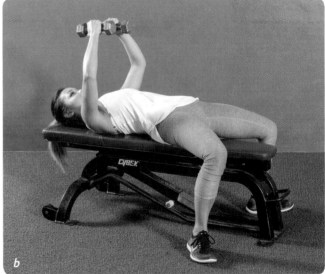

MID CABLE FLY

This move targets the chest muscles, particularly the middle portion.

Chest Category 4

START

Grasp the handles of a pulley attached to a cable apparatus, and adjust the height so that the handles are at just below shoulder level. Face away from the apparatus. Stand with your feet about shoulder-width apart, with one foot in front of the other, your torso bent slightly forward at the waist, and your arms slightly bent and held out to the sides so that they are approximately parallel to the floor.

MOVEMENT

Keeping your upper body motionless and your core muscles tight, pull both handles across your body, creating a semicircular movement. Bring your hands together at the level of your chest, and squeeze your chest muscles so that you feel a contraction in the cleavage area. Then reverse the direction, allowing your hands to return along the same path to the start position.

EXPERT TIP

Your elbows should remain slightly bent and fixed throughout the move; don't flex or extend them at any time. This error effectively makes the exercise a pressing movement rather than a fly.

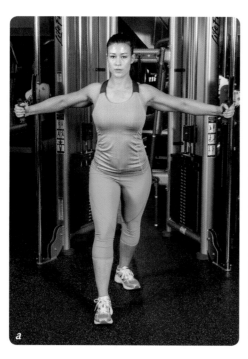 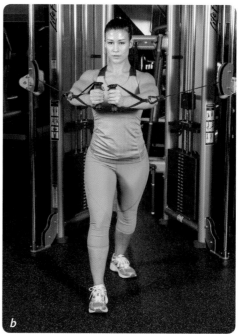

PEC DECK FLY

This move targets the chest muscles, particularly the middle portion.

Chest Category 4

START

Grasp the handles of a pec deck machine, palms facing one another. Your back should remain immobile throughout the movement.

MOVEMENT

Simultaneously press both handles together, allowing your hands to gently touch directly in front of your chest. Contract your pectoral muscles and then reverse direction, returning to the start position.

EXPERT TIP

There are several types of pec deck units. They all accomplish the same task, so use whatever version is available.

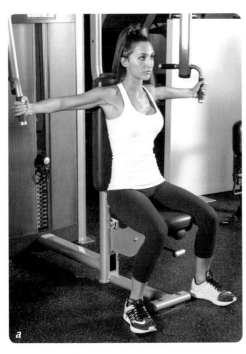
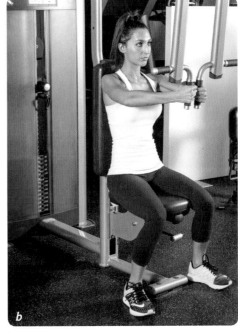

ABDOMINAL EXERCISES

Exercises for the abdominals are divided into the following three categories (see table 5.3):

- Category 1 comprises exercises involving spinal flexion.
- Category 2 comprises exercises involving lateral flexion or rotation.
- Category 3 comprises exercises that statically challenge the abdominal musculature.

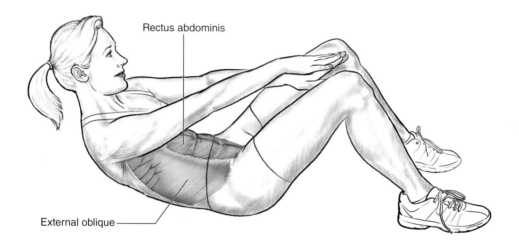

Rectus abdominis

External oblique

Table 5.3 Abdominal Exercises by Category

Category 1	Category 2	Category 3
Crunch	Bicycle crunch	Plank
Reverse crunch	Cable kneeling twisting rope crunch	Side bridge
Hanging knee raise	Cable side bend	Antirotation press
Barbell kneeling rollout	Cable woodchop	Long-lever posterior-tilt plank
Stability ball crunch	Stability ball side crunch	
Cable kneeling rope crunch		
Toe touch		

CRUNCH

This move targets the abs with a focus on the upper abdominal region.

Abdominal Category 1

START

Lie faceup on the floor with your knees bent and your feet planted. Press your low back into the floor and fold your hands across your chest.

MOVEMENT

Keeping your low back fixed to the floor, raise your shoulders up and forward as high as possible. Feel a contraction in your abdominal muscles and then reverse direction, returning to the start position.

EXPERT TIPS

- Don't allow your upper back to touch the floor when lowering; doing so reduces tension in the abs.
- If the move becomes easy, hold a weighted object (such as a dumbbell or medicine ball) against your chest.
- Never place your hands behind your head; this facilitates pulling on the neck muscles, which can lead to injury.

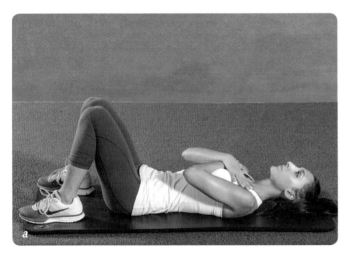 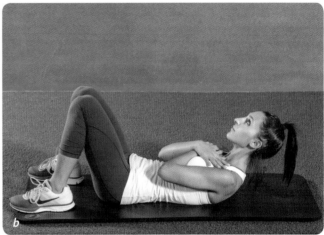

REVERSE CRUNCH

This move targets the abs with a focus on the lower abdominal region.

Abdominal Category 1

START

Lie supine on the floor with your hands at your sides. Curl your knees into your midsection and lift your butt so that it is slightly off the floor.

MOVEMENT

Keeping your upper back pressed into the floor, raise your butt as high as possible so that your pelvis tilts toward your chest. Contract your abs and then reverse direction, returning to the start position.

EXPERT TIPS

- Don't just push your butt up in the air. Rather, focus on pulling your pelvis backward so that it approaches your belly button. This forces the lower portion of the abs to do more of the work. It's a short range of motion that, when done properly, really hits the target musculature.
- Don't allow your butt to touch the floor when lowering; doing so reduces tension in the abs.
- If the move becomes easy, you can place a medicine ball between your thighs.

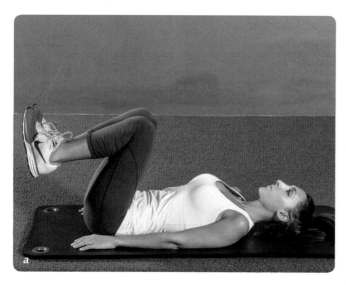
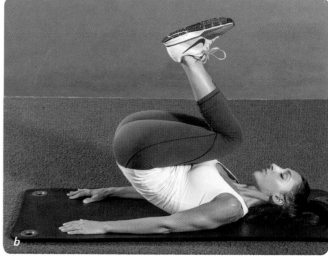

HANGING KNEE RAISE

This move targets the abs, particularly the lower abdominal region.

Abdominal Category 1

START

Grasp a chinning bar with a shoulder-width grip, bend your knees, and stabilize your torso.

MOVEMENT

Keeping your knees bent, raise your thighs, lifting your butt so that your pelvis tilts toward your abdomen. Contract your abs and then reverse direction, returning your legs to the start position. For increased intensity, straighten your legs while performing the move.

EXPERT TIPS

- Focus on pulling your pelvis up and back so that it approaches your belly button. This forces the lower portion of the abs to do more of the work.
- If you have trouble holding your body weight, consider using hanging ab straps.
- Keep your upper torso motionless throughout the move; don't swing to complete a repetition.

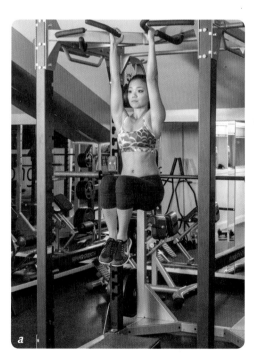
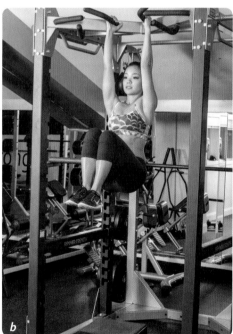

BARBELL KNEELING ROLLOUT

This move targets the abs.

Abdominal Category 1

START

Load a pair of small plates (5-pounders work well [about 2 kg]) onto the ends of a barbell. Grasp the middle of the bar with an overhand, shoulder-width grip, and kneel down so that your shoulders are directly over the bar.

MOVEMENT

Keeping your knees fixed on the floor and your arms taut, roll the bar forward as far as comfortably possible without allowing your body to touch the floor. Reverse direction by forcefully contracting your abs, returning along the same path to the start position.

EXPERT TIP

The contraction happens as you pull back to the start position (the rollout stretches the abs), so focus on actively contracting the musculature as you pull the bar inward.

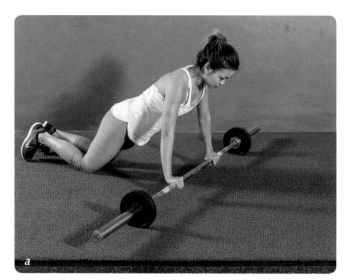 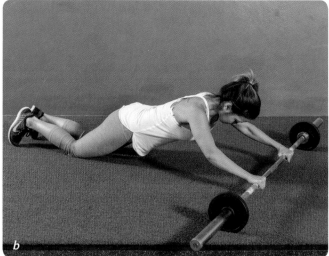

STABILITY BALL CRUNCH

This move targets the abdominals.

Abdominal Category 1

START

Sit on top of the ball with your feet shoulder-width apart. Walk your feet forward until your low back is firmly supported. Place your hands on your chest and lower your upper back and shoulders onto the ball.

MOVEMENT

Lift your upper back and shoulders off the ball as far as comfortably possible. Contract your abs and return along the same path to the start position.

EXPERT TIPS

- Sitting higher on the ball (i.e., butt on top of the ball) makes the exercise more difficult, whereas sitting lower on the ball makes it easier.
- Your low back should remain on the ball at all times. Lifting your low back engages the hip flexors, reducing stress to the target muscles.
- Keep your hips anchored so that you move over the ball and the ball does not roll under you.
- If the move becomes easy, hold a weighted object (such as a dumbbell or medicine ball) against your chest.

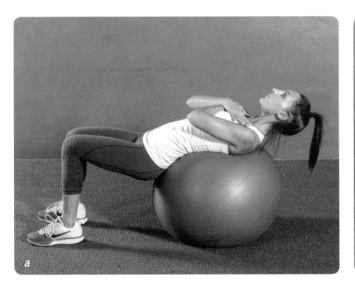
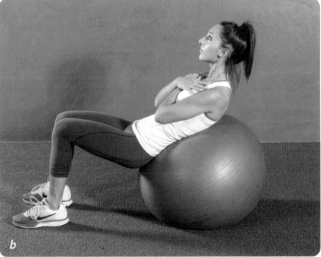

CABLE KNEELING ROPE CRUNCH

This move targets abdominals, with a focus on the upper portion.

Abdominal Category 1

START

Begin by facing a high pulley attached to a cable apparatus and then kneel down, sitting back on your heels. Grasp the ends of a rope attached to the pulley, and keep your elbows next to your ears and your torso upright.

MOVEMENT

Keeping your low back immobile, curl your shoulders down, bringing your elbows down toward your knees. Contract your abs and then uncurl your body, returning to the start position.

EXPERT TIP

Curl only from your upper torso; your hips should remain fixed throughout the move. This maintains tension in the abs.

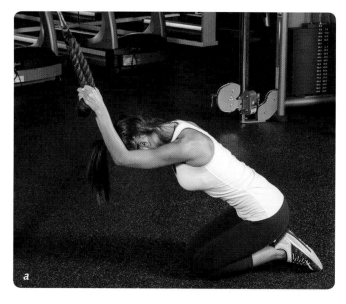
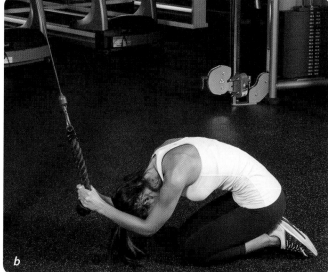

TOE TOUCH

This move targets the abs with a focus on the upper abdominal region.

Abdominal Category 1

START

Lie faceup on the floor with your arms and legs straight in the air, perpendicular to your body.

MOVEMENT

Keeping your low back pressed to the floor, curl your torso up and forward, raising your hands as close to your toes as possible. Contract your abs and then reverse direction, returning to the start position.

EXPERT TIPS

- Your lumbar region should remain fixed throughout the move; only your upper back should rise off the floor.
- Keep your head stable at all times; any unwanted movement can cause injury to the cervical spine.
- For added intensity, hold a weighted object (such as a dumbbell or medicine ball) in your hands.

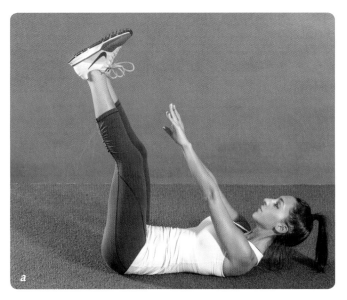

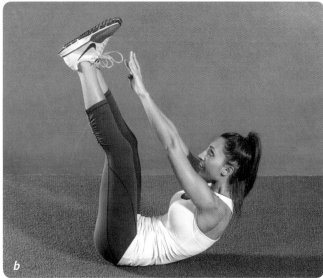

BICYCLE CRUNCH

This move targets the abs.

Abdominal Category 2

START

Lie faceup on the floor with your legs bent at a 90-degree angle. Ball your hands into fists and place them at your ears.

MOVEMENT

Bring your left knee up toward your right elbow and try to make contact between the two. As you return your left leg and right elbow to the start position, bring your right leg toward your left elbow in the same manner. Continue this movement, alternating between right and left sides as if pedaling a bike.

EXPERT TIPS

- Never place your hands behind your head; this facilitates pulling on the neck muscles, which can lead to injury.
- People commonly speed up on this move; avoid the temptation. As with all exercises, perform this one in a smooth, controlled manner for optimal results.

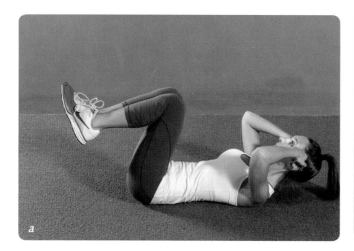 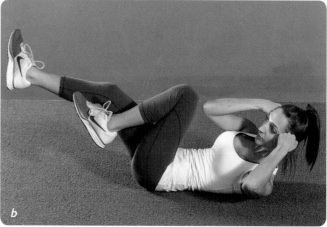

CABLE KNEELING TWISTING ROPE CRUNCH

This move targets the abdominals and the obliques.

Abdominal Category 2

START

Begin by facing a high pulley attached to a cable apparatus, and then kneel down and sit back on your heels. Grasp the ends of a rope attached to the pulley, and keep your elbows next to your ears and your torso upright.

MOVEMENT

Keeping your low back immobile, curl your shoulders down, twisting your body to the left as you bring your elbows toward your left knee. Contract your abs and then uncurl your body, returning to the start position. Alternate between twisting to the right and to the left for the desired number of repetitions.

EXPERT TIP

Curl only from your upper torso; your hips should remain fixed throughout the move. This maintains tension in the target muscles.

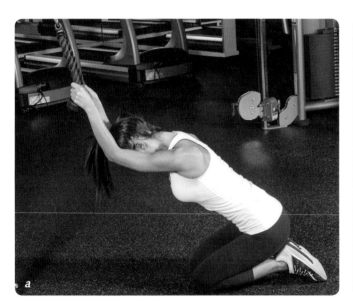
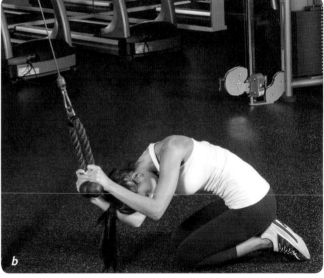

CABLE SIDE BEND

This move targets the obliques.

Abdominal Category 2

START

Grasp a loop handle attached to the low pulley of a cable apparatus with your right hand. With your right side facing the machine, take a small step away from the machine so that there is tension in the cable. Keep your feet shoulder-width apart, your right arm straight, your torso erect, and your knees slightly bent.

MOVEMENT

Keeping your core tight, bend your torso as far to the left as possible without discomfort. Contract your obliques and then return along the same path to the start position. After performing the desired number of reps, repeat on the opposite side.

EXPERT TIPS

- The movement should take place solely at your waist; your hips shouldn't move at all during the move.
- Your upper body should remain in the same plane at all times; don't sway forward or backward.

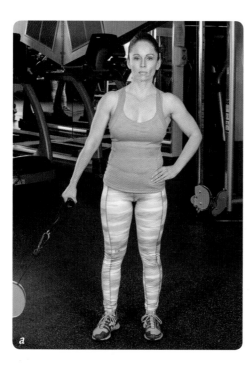 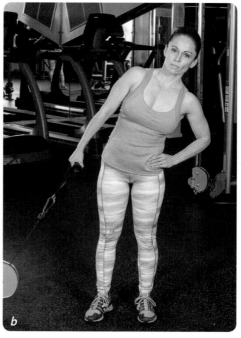

CABLE WOODCHOP

This move targets the obliques.

Abdominal Category 2

START

Grasp the ends of a rope attached to a cable pulley apparatus. If possible, adjust the cable so that it is at chest height (if the machine is not adjustable, you can perform the move from the high- or low-pulley positions). Keep your feet shoulder-width apart, your torso erect, and your knees slightly bent. Position your body so that your right side faces the machine, and extend your arms as far as comfortably possible across your body to the right.

MOVEMENT

Keeping your lower body stable, pull the rope up and across your torso to the left with a motion as if you were chopping wood. Contract your obliques and then return along the same path to the start position. After performing the desired number of reps, repeat on the opposite side.

EXPERT TIP

To keep constant tension on the obliques, make sure the action takes place at your waist, not your hips.

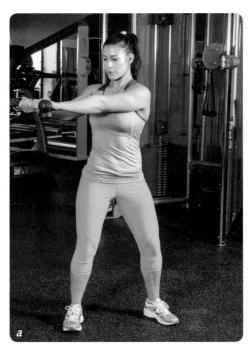
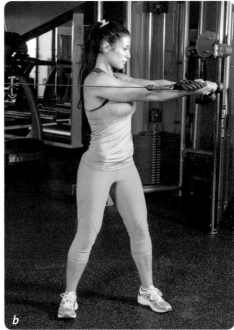

STABILITY BALL SIDE CRUNCH

This move targets the obliques.

Abdominal Category 2

START

Lie sideways on the top of a stability ball with your feet planted firmly on the floor. Place your fingertips by your temples and your elbows wide of your body, and lower your bottom elbow as far as comfortably possible.

MOVEMENT

Keeping your fingertips pressed to your temples, raise your top elbow so that your trunk laterally flexes as far as possible. Contract your obliques and then return along the same path to the start position. After performing the desired number of reps, repeat on the opposite side.

EXPERT TIP

If you have trouble maintaining stability, buttress your feet up against the bottom of a wall for support.

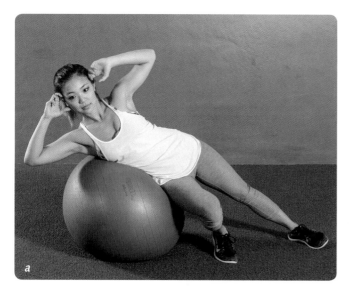

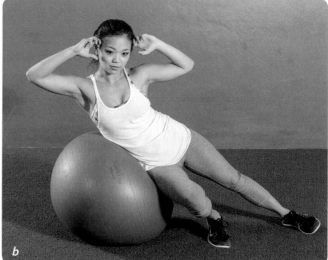

PLANK

This move statically targets the abs.

Abdominal Category 3

START

Lie facedown on the floor with your feet together and your spine and pelvis neutrally aligned. Your hands should be balled into fists and kept in a neutral position (i.e., thumbs up and little fingers on the floor) with elbows aligned below your shoulders.

MOVEMENT

Lift your body up on your forearms and toes, keeping your body as straight as possible. Maintain this position for as long as possible, and challenge yourself to maintain longer periods in the plank position.

EXPERT TIPS

- Use your core strength to keep your body rigid; don't allow any part of your body to sag at any time.
- Use a stopwatch to time yourself.
- If you can hold the position for longer than 30 seconds, switch to a more challenging version such as the long-lever posterior-tilt plank, or use an unstable surface such as a stability ball.

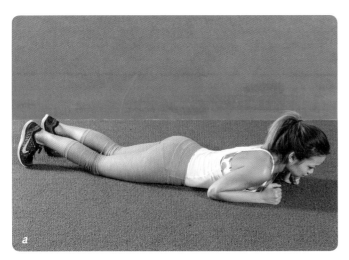
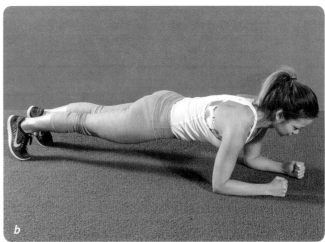

SIDE BRIDGE

This move targets the abdominals, particularly the obliques.

Abdominal Category 3

START

Lie on your left side with your legs straight, your left forearm on the floor, and your feet stacked one on top of the other.

MOVEMENT

Lift your hips off the floor, and place your free hand on your opposite hip. Hold this position for as long as possible, and then repeat on the opposite side.

EXPERT TIPS

- Use your core strength to keep your body rigid; don't allow any part of your body to sag at any time.
- Balance on the sides of your feet, not the soles.
- Aim to work up to a 30-second hold or more.
- Use a stopwatch to time yourself.
- For added intensity, perform the move on an unstable device such as a BOSU trainer or a small stability ball.
- For a greater level of difficulty, you can modify the move by placing your hand on the floor and straightening your arm to move into the bridge position.

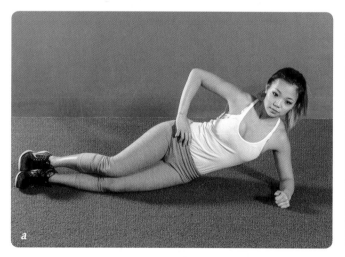
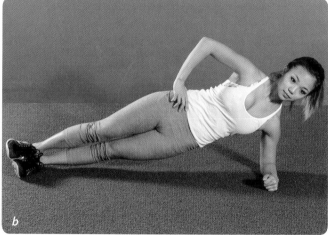

ANTIROTATION PRESS

This move targets the abdominals.

Abdominal Category 3

START

With both hands, grasp a loop handle attached to a cable apparatus set at the height of your midsection. Rotate your body so that your right side is facing away from the weight stack, and hold your hands in front of your abdomen.

MOVEMENT

Keeping your body stable and your back in a neutral position, push your hands straight out in front of you, extending your arms forward. Hold this position for several seconds and then return to the start position. After performing the desired number of reps, repeat on the opposite side.

EXPERT TIP

You can perform this exercise from a half-kneeling position in which one knee is on the floor and the other leg is bent at a 90-degree angle with the foot flat on the floor.

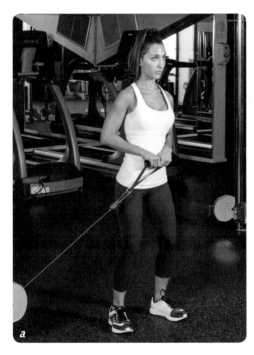
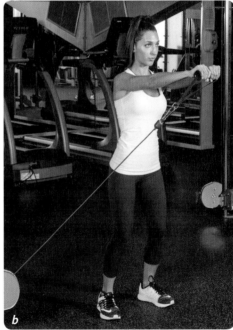

LONG-LEVER POSTERIOR-TILT PLANK

This move targets the abs. An advanced variation of the traditional plank, it substantially increases activation of the musculature.

Abdominal Category 3

START

Lie facedown on the floor with your feet together and your spine and pelvis neutrally aligned. Your hands should be balled into fists and kept in a neutral position (i.e., thumbs up and little fingers on the floor). The elbows should be spaced approximately 6 inches (15 cm) apart at nose level.

MOVEMENT

Lift your body up on your forearms and toes so that your elbows are at an approximately 100-degree angle and the torso and lower extremities form a straight line with the lumbar spine in a neutral position. Contract your gluteals as strongly as possible while attempting to draw your pubic bone toward your belly button and your tailbone toward your feet. Hold this position as long as possible while continuing to attempt to maximally contract your glutes.

EXPERT TIPS

- To heighten the level of difficulty, move your elbows closer to your eyes, which increases the lever length.
- Don't allow your hips to drop or sag at any point during performance.
- Aim to work up to a 30-second hold or more.
- Use a stopwatch to time yourself.

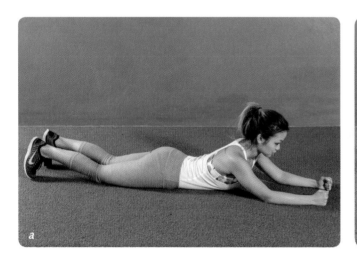
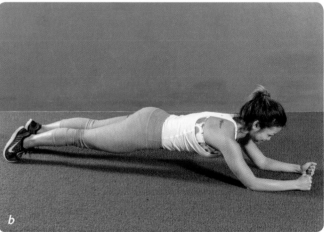

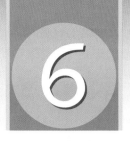

Warm-Up

To prepare your body for the demands of intense exercise, you should warm up prior to your lifting session. The warm-up contains two basic components: a general warm-up and a specific warm-up. Here's what you need to know about each component for a safe, effective workout.

GENERAL WARM-UP

The general warm-up is a brief bout of low-intensity, large muscle-group, aerobic-type exercise. The objective is to elevate your core temperature and increase blood flow, which in turn enhances the speed of nerve impulses, increases nutrient delivery to working muscles and the removal of waste by-products, and facilitates oxygen release from hemoglobin and myoglobin.

A direct correlation exists between muscle temperature and exercise performance: When a muscle is warm, it can achieve a better contraction. As a rule, the higher a muscle's temperature is (within a safe physiological range), the better its contractility. And because better contractility translates into greater force production, you'll ultimately achieve better muscular development.

What's more, an elevated core temperature diminishes a joint's resistance to flow (viscosity). This is accomplished via the uptake of synovial fluid, which is secreted from the synovial membrane to lubricate the joint. The net effect is an increase in range of motion and improved joint-related resiliency. Better yet, these factors combine to reduce the risk of a training-related injury.

Suffice it to say that the general warm-up is an important part of a workout.

Virtually any cardiorespiratory activity can be used for the general warm-up. Exercises on equipment such as stationary bikes, stair climbers, and treadmills are fine choices, as are most calisthenic-type exercises (e.g., jumping jacks, burpees). Choose whatever activity you desire as long as the basic objective is met.

The intensity for the general warm-up should be low. To estimate intensity of training, I like to use a rating of perceived exertion (RPE) scale. My preference is the category-ratio RPE scale, which grades perceived effort on a scale from 0 to 10 (0 is lying on your couch, and 10 is an all-out sprint). Aim for an RPE of around 5, which for most people is a moderate walk or slow jog. You can use the talk test as an intensity gauge. With this method, you base intensity on your ability to carry on a conversation; if you have to pause to take a breath while speaking a sentence, you're working too hard.

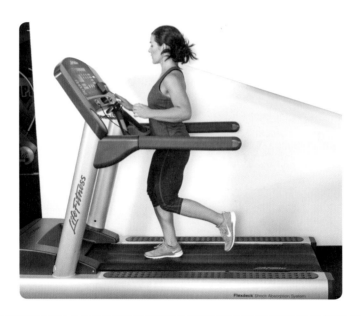

Virtually any large-muscle group aerobic exercise can be used for the general warm-up.

Five to ten minutes is all you need for the general warm-up—just enough to break a light sweat. Your resources should not be taxed, nor should you feel tired or out of breath either during or after performance. If so, cut back on the intensity. Remember, the goal here is merely to warm your body tissues and accelerate blood flow—not to achieve cardiorespiratory benefits or reduce body fat.

SPECIFIC WARM-UP

The specific warm-up can be considered an extension of the general warm-up. By using exercises that are similar to the activities in the workout, the specific warm-up enhances neuromuscular efficiency for the exercise you are about to perform. In essence, your body gets to rehearse the movements before you perform them at a high level of intensity, translating into better performance during your working sets.

To optimize transfer of training, the exercises in the specific warm-up should mimic the movements in the workout as closely as possible. For example, if you are going to perform a bench press, the specific warm-up would ideally include light sets of bench presses. A viable alternative would be to perform push-ups because the movement pattern is similar to that of a bench press, although the specificity, and thus transfer, would not be as great as with light sets of the given movement. Always stop specific warm-up sets well short of fatigue. The object is not to fatigue your muscles, but rather to get a feel for the exercise so that you're physically and mentally prepared for intense training.

The specific warm-up is particularly important when training in low-repetition ranges (~ five reps or fewer). I recommend at least a couple of specific warm-up sets per exercise during low-rep training. As a general rule, the first set should be performed at ~40 to 50 percent of 1RM; and the second set, at ~60 to 70 percent of 1RM. Six to eight reps is all you need in these sets—any more is superfluous and potentially counterproductive. Following the specific warm-up, you should be ready and able to plow into your working sets.

The need for specific warm-up sets in medium- to high-rep-range training remains questionable. I recently collaborated on a study that investigated the effects of a warm-up on the ability to carry out repetitions to failure at 80 percent of 1RM (a weight that allows performance of about eight reps) in the squat, bench press, and arm curl (Ribeiro et al., 2014). The verdict: Warming up showed no beneficial effects on the number of repetitions performed in medium- to high-rep-range training nor in a measure called the fatigue index, which is a formula that assesses the decline in the number of repetitions across the first and last sets of each exercise.

At face value these results suggest that warming up is pretty much useless prior to submaximal resistance training. Despite the currently held belief that a specific warm-up enhances exercise performance, no benefits were seen when compared to no warm-up at all. Intuitively, this seems to make sense given that the initial repetitions of a submaximal lifts are in effect their own specific warm-up, and increasing core temperature might be superfluous from a performance standpoint when multiple reps are performed.

It should be noted, however, that we found a slight advantage to performing a specific warm-up prior to the squat (although results did not rise to statistical significance); the specific warm-up prior to the biceps curl seemed to be somewhat detrimental. Thus, more complex movement patterns seem to benefit from the practice effect of a specific warm-up, although this would be of no value prior to simple exercises.

Taking the evidence into account, here's my recommendation: When performing medium-rep-range work (8 to 12 reps per set), perform a specific warm-up prior to multijoint free weight exercises. One set at about 50 percent of 1RM is all you need to obtain any potential benefits.

Specific warm-up sets are not necessary when training with high reps (15+ reps per set). In this instance, because you're already using light weights, the initial repetitions of each working set serve as rehearsal reps. What's more, performance of warm-up sets is counterproductive to the goal of maximizing training density to bring about desired metabolic adaptations.

WHAT ABOUT STRETCHING?

Static stretching is commonly included as part of a prelifting warm-up. This method of flexibility training involves moving a joint through its range of motion to the point where you feel slight discomfort, and then holding the position for a period of time (generally about 30 seconds). Most protocols involve performing several sets of static holds and then moving on to stretches for other muscles. It's commonly believed that the addition of stretches to a warm-up further reduces injury risk while enhancing physical performance.

In recent years, however, the benefits of preexercise static stretching have come under scrutiny. A large body of research shows that the practice does not decrease injury risk (Thacker et al., 2004). Yes, improving flexibility can conceivably help in injury prevention. Tight muscles have been implicated as a cause of training-related injury, and improving flexibility can reduce this possibility. Because a stretching exercise improves range of motion, including it in an exercise program can enhance overall workout safety. However, the benefits are not specific to stretching prior to training. All that matters is achieving adequate range of motion to properly carry out exercise performance.

The most important consideration here is to make sure your muscles are warm before performing static stretches. This reduces joint viscosity, ensuring that muscles and connective tissue are sufficiently prepped to endure passive or active lengthening.

So you might be thinking, Why not include some basic stretches after the general warm-up? After all, your core temperature is elevated and joint viscosity is reduced. What's the harm, right?

Interestingly, evidence shows that static stretching performed before a workout can have a detrimental impact on exercise performance. This is most applicable to activities requiring high force output, such as heavy resistance training. The primary theory proposed to account for these performance decrements is a decrease in musculotendinous stiffness. The musculotendinous unit (the muscle and its associated tendons) is responsible for generating force to carry out movement. Like an overstretched rubber band, the musculotendinous unit with increased laxity following stretching impairs force transmission. The upshot is a reduced capacity to lift a given load.

However, caution needs to be used when applying this research to a lifting session. First, most of the studies in question used excessive stretching protocols, in some cases upwards of 30 minutes stretching a single joint! Most preworkout stretching routines involve only a few minutes per joint, and it's highly questionable whether such brief stretching bouts have any performance-related detriments. Moreover, the vast majority of research on the topic is specific to high-strength and high-power activities. Whether negative effects are associated when training with medium- to high-rep schemes remains speculative.

Given the uncertainty of evidence, you're best off performing static stretches immediately after your workout. Your body is already warm from engaging in intense exercise, and it generally feels good to cool down by elongating muscles that have been repeatedly contracted. Some research even shows that postworkout stretching may alleviate delayed-onset muscle soreness (see the sidebar What Causes Muscle Soreness After a Workout?), although the extent of the reduction probably isn't all that meaningful (Henschke & Lin, 2011).

If you want to include some flexibility work prior to lifting, consider dynamic stretches: slow, controlled movements taken through their full range of motion. Examples are arm swings, shoulder circles, high steps, and hip twists. Choose dynamic stretches that are specific to the joint actions being trained in your workout. Perform several sets for each dynamic stretch, attempting to move the body segment farther and farther in a comfortable range with each set.

Contrary to popular belief, you don't have to include a stretching component in your regular routine. Increased flexibility results in decreased joint stability. Being too flexible, therefore, actually increases injury risk. Thus, stretch only those joints that are tight, and avoid any additional flexibility exercise for those that already have adequate range of motion to carry out your required activities of daily living.

Moreover, it's important to note that resistance training in itself actually improves flexibility. Provided that you train through a complete range of motion, multiset lifting protocols produce similar increases in flexibility to those seen with static stretching routines (Morton et al., 2011). In essence, resistance training is an active form of flexibility training whereby a muscle is contracted and then immediately lengthened. When performed on a regular basis, it can keep you mobile and limber. We can therefore put to rest the myth that lifting slows you down and binds you up!

What Causes Muscle Soreness After a Workout?

Following an intense workout, many people feel sore in their trained muscles. This phenomenon, called delayed-onset muscle soreness (DOMS), generally develops a day or two after training and can last 72 hours or more. The soreness can be mild or very severe, depending on a number of factors including genetics, muscle action, and intensity of effort, amongst others.

The cause of DOMS is often misunderstood. Contrary to popular belief, it is totally unrelated to a buildup of lactic acid. The truth is, lactate is rapidly cleared from muscles following a workout. Within an hour or two postexercise, it is either completely oxidized or used for glycogen resynthesis. Because DOMS doesn't manifest until at least 24 hours after a training session, it follows that lactic acid cannot play a part in its origin.

So what causes DOMS? It's actually a product of damage to muscle tissue. Intense exercise produces small microtears in the working muscle fibers, primarily as a result of eccentric activity (i.e., lengthening a muscle against tension). These microtears allow calcium to escape from the muscles, disrupting their intracellular balance. Metabolic waste is produced, and that interacts with the free nerve endings surrounding the damaged fibers, resulting in localized pain and stiffness.

In response, white blood cells migrate to the site of injury, generating free radicals that further exacerbate the sensation of pain. The discomfort can last for several days or even up to a week, depending on the extent of muscle damage.

So, don't blame lactic acid buildup for making you sore after a workout. It's merely a sign that you've worked the fibers in an accustomed fashion. If you experience DOMS, the best thing you can do is stay active in the postexercise period, thereby enhancing blood flow to the affected area. This will expedite the delivery of nutrients to the muscles, accelerating the rate of their repair and reducing the associated discomfort.

Break-In Phase

One of the biggest mistakes fitness newbies make is attempting to follow the workout routine of their favorite physique competitor. This is completely understandable. It's only natural to assume that what works for her should work for you as well. After all, she must know a thing or two about exercise program design to be in such amazing shape, right?

Here's the rub: A workout program must be initiated in a systematic fashion, taking into account your particular needs and abilities. Elite physique athletes have spent years acclimating their bodies to the demands of intense training. If you lack the requisite training experience, advanced exercise programs are likely to overwhelm your recuperative abilities and rapidly bring about a state of overtraining. Not only will you fail to get the results you desire, but you'll also actually regress in your efforts.

The break-in phase is for those who are new to resistance training or coming off an extended layoff. If you fall into either of these categories, I highly recommend starting here. If you're a seasoned lifter, feel free to skip this chapter and proceed to more advanced phases of the program. Before doing so, however, make sure that you have honestly assessed your ability to handle the stresses of intense exercise. Engaging in a rigorous training program, as required in future phases of the program, before you're physically and mentally ready is bound to leave you overtrained and unable to derive intended benefits. This will set back your progress, potentially for weeks if not months. So if you have any doubt as to whether you're prepared for the program, err on the side of caution and start with the break-in phase.

Better safe than sorry.

To clarify the goal of the break-in phase, I like to use an analogy that compares body sculpting to building a house. The foundation is what the structure of a house rests on. Without a solid foundation, the entire house crumbles. Just as a builder can't erect the frame of the house before a foundation is in place, you must develop a strong foundation of muscle on which to build. To quote a popular fitness axiom: You can't shape what you don't have.

And it's not just your muscles that need to be developed; the supporting connective tissue must be considered as well. Strengthening these tissues is important for the proper transmission of resistance forces and the maintenance of joint health. Remember, a chain is only as strong as its weakest link.

Foundational training is also essential for developing the requisite skills to perform basic exercise movements. To properly target your muscles, you first must be able to carry out exercises under precise control. If you fail to master lifting performance, your muscular development will suffer.

As a general rule, you should remain in this phase for approximately two to three months. If you're new to training, you'll probably be on the higher side of this estimate, whereas if you're returning from a layoff, a few weeks may be all you need to get back on track. When in doubt, err on the side of caution. It's better to continue with the break-in phase for a few extra weeks than to find yourself without the structural foundation you need to reap optimal results from ensuing phases.

What follows is the protocol for the break-in phase as well as a sample routine that illustrates how to put it all together.

COMPOSITION OF THE ROUTINE

The break-in phase employs a total-body routine in which you work all the major muscle groups during every session. This approach results in frequent stimulation of your neuromuscular system, which facilitates early-phase motor learning. The initial stages of training are characterized by ingraining neuromotor patterns for the exercises performed; muscle development is minimal during these first few weeks. This is a process of integration between your brain and your muscles whereby your body figures out how to carry out movements in the most efficient manner possible.

Three neural mechanisms govern your ability to exert force: recruitment, rate coding, and synchronization. Recruitment refers to the ability of your nervous system to activate motor units; rate coding refers to the frequency by which nerve impulses are stimulated during a lift; and synchronization refers to the coordinated timing between muscle fibers (called intramuscular coordination) or between synergists (called intermuscular coordination). Repeated performance of the exercises optimizes all three components, facilitating smooth, efficient movement patterns. The result is an enhanced level of neuromuscular control whereby the proper muscles can produce the proper amount of force in the proper amount of time for a given movement. Once you are proficient, you can focus on engaging the target muscles to exert maximal force.

FREQUENCY

In this phase you train three days a week on nonconsecutive days. Generally speaking, you need about 48 hours to recover between intense workouts for the same muscle group. This corresponds to the time course for muscle protein synthesis, which lasts approximately a couple of days following a lifting session. A Monday/Wednesday/Friday or Tuesday/Thursday/Saturday schedule is typical. If you miss a day, simply train on the following day and resume the alternate-day approach. For example, if you are on the Monday/Wednesday/Friday schedule and can't make the Wednesday session, then work out Thursday and Saturday instead. The following week you can resume your normal training schedule. The most important thing is getting in the required amount of weekly workouts if at all possible. Remember, repetition of performance is what ingrains movement patterns. Dedication during the initial stages of training is especially vital for long-term results.

EXERCISES

Given that all major muscles are worked in a session, you perform just one exercise per muscle group. This keeps the overall volume manageable for a given training bout. Recall that excessive volume leads to an overtrained state, which hampers progress and impairs health. You are especially susceptible to overtraining during the early stages of training because your body has not yet adapted to the stresses of intense lifting. Thus, you need to manage your volume carefully so that it does not exceed your recuperative abilities.

The focus here should be on multijoint exercises. These movements are highly efficient because they work large amounts of muscle in a single exercise—an important consideration when the number of exercises performed per muscle group is restricted. What's more, multijoint exercises generally involve greater engagement of the all-important stabilizer muscles. For example, the primary movers in a barbell back squat are the quads and glutes with dynamic assistance from the hamstrings and calves. However, numerous stabilizers must help out to maintain an erect posture, keep the barbell along the shoulders, and prevent swaying from side to side. Muscles such as the erector spinae, rhomboids, and external rotators act in an isometric fashion to accomplish this task. Developing these muscles is essential to build the foundation discussed earlier that facilitates development later on.

Exercise selection is highly limited in the break-in phase: The same basic movements are performed during each session. Although this might seem rudimentary and perhaps a tad boring, it is an important conditioning strategy. Remember that muscular adaptations during the initial stages of training are primarily neural; muscle hypertrophy (increases in the size of the muscles) is minimal at this point. Your body is getting used to new movement patterns, finding the most economical way to perform the exercises. Concentrating on a limited number of exercises expedites skill acquisition, fostering the development of coordinated motor programs.

There are no must-do exercises. If an exercise doesn't feel right to you or if you are having difficulty picking up the movement pattern, switch to a different exercise of your liking. Just make sure that the substituted movement is similar to the one in question. I've made the process of substitution simple by segmenting exercise descriptions into categories based on movement patterns for each muscle group. If you swap out an exercise, just choose another from the same category and you will ensure a balanced workout.

Note that this phase does not include direct work for the upper arms and calves. The reason is that training time is limited and all your energies during this phase need to be focused on exercises that work as much muscle as possible. Don't worry, though. These muscles will get ample stimulation during compound exercises for the upper and lower body; presses and rows heavily involve the arm muscles, and squats and lunges engage musculature in the lower legs. Besides, research shows that adding direct arm exercises to a routine consisting of multijoint movements does little to increase muscle growth in the biceps and triceps during the first few months of training (Gentil et al., 2013). And rest assured, you'll blitz these muscle groups during the ensuing phases of the program to optimize their development.

SETS

You perform four sets per exercise during this phase. Although some evidence suggests that a single set is sufficient for substantially increasing muscle and strength over the course of the first few months of training, multiple sets have been shown to be superior in this regard (Krieger, 2009, 2010). Just as important, if not more so, is the fact that the additional sets provide extra practice time on the given exercises. The repeated performance of movements is what ingrains motor patterns so that execution is carried out in a smooth, controlled fashion. More practice equals faster results.

REPETITIONS

In the break-in phase, you adhere to a moderate- to high-repetition range, targeting 10 to 15 reps per set. Like using multiple sets, performing more reps provides more practice time, which improves your neuromuscular control during each exercise. In addition, it relieves you from having to generate high levels of force, thereby allowing you to focus on developing proper exercise technique. Understand that the sole objective in this phase is to build a foundation on which to sculpt your muscles. Once you learn the basic movements, muscle development will soon follow.

REST INTERVALS

You should take approximately two-minutes rests between sets. This is a sufficient amount of time to recover your strength reserves, particularly given that the level of effort is not that high in this phase of the program. There's no reason to spend additional time in the gym sitting around between sets if it's not necessary. That said, if you feel you need extra intra-set rest, take it. The most important consideration here is to be sufficiently recuperated to channel all of your energies into performing the next set without compromising form.

INTENSITY OF EFFORT

The weights you use should be moderately challenging during the first several weeks of training and then progressively increase over the ensuing weeks. Again, the initial goal here is to develop neuromuscular control; generating high levels of force is not a concern. Moreover, form tends to break down as you approach muscular failure, especially if you have not completely ingrained neuromuscular patterns for the exercise.

As the weeks go by, you should progressively increase your level of effort so that, after a month or so, you are beginning to push to the point of muscular failure. But again, don't do so at the expense of good form. Not only is such a practice detrimental to the objective of this phase, but you also increase the potential for an injury that can derail your training efforts.

Here's how things should play out using the reps-to-failure (RTF) scale from chapter 2 to estimate effort (see table 2.1):

- Weeks 1 and 2: Your level of effort during the first couple of weeks should correspond to a 4 on the RTF for all sets. This equates to selecting a weight that allows you to achieve the target rep range with approximately four or more reps in reserve. Challenge to your muscles will be minimal.

- Weeks 3 and 4: Your level of effort should increase so that you're at a 3 on the RTF scale on the first two sets of each exercise. This equates to achieving the target rep range with approximately three reps in reserve. The final two sets should correspond to a 2 on the RTF scale, meaning that you're stopping approximately two reps short of failure. At this point, the sets will be fairly challenging; you'll start to struggle a bit on the last rep or so.

- Weeks 5+: Increase your level of effort further so that you're at an RTF of 3 on the first set, 2 on the second set, 1 on the third set, and 0 on the fourth and final set. This means that you take the last set to the point of momentary muscular failure (i.e., performance of another rep is not possible).

Table 7.1 summarizes the break-in phase protocol. A sample routine is provided in table 7.2. These routines are intended to serve as a basic template for constructing your workouts. Modify specific exercises according to your needs and abilities.

Table 7.1 Summary of the Break-In Phase

Training variable	Protocol
Sets	4 per exercise
Repetitions	10-15
Rest intervals	2 min
Frequency	3 days a week

Table 7.2   Sample Break-In Phase Routine

WEEK ONE					
Monday, Wednesday, Friday					
Exercise	Exercise photo	Sets	Repetitions	Rest interval	Page number
Dumbbell chest press		4	10-15	2 min	125
Dumbbell single-arm row		4	10-15	2 min	109
Military press		4	10-15	2 min	24
Barbell back squat		4	10-15	2 min	64
Dumbbell lunge		4	10-15	2 min	69
Dumbbell stiff-leg deadlift		4	10-15	2 min	82

Basic Training Phase

If you've completed the break-in phase, congrats! You've officially graduated from newbie status. Now it's time to step things up a bit.

The basic training phase is for those who either have completed the break-in phase or have some lifting experience but have been training for less than a year. This phase is essentially an extension of the break-in phase and is designed to further develop a sound structure to your physique. It's an intermediate-level program that builds on what you've accomplished to help you transition to more advanced training practices.

To appreciate the objective of this phase, let's again revisit the analogy of building a house. In the break-in phase you acquired basic neuromuscular skills and initiated the development of your muscles and connective tissue. This provided a solid foundation on which to build.

Your aim now is akin to erecting the frame of the house. The frame provides the supporting structure that defines the house's overall appearance. It allows you to add things such as hardwood floors, marble countertops, and other accoutrements that give the house character. From a body-sculpting standpoint, erecting a frame equates to further conditioning bodily systems to the demands of intense training. Your neuromuscular system must become more efficient so that exercise performance is second nature. Moreover, your immune system must be able to respond to the demands of intense exercise to facilitate optimal recuperation and remodeling. Once you've achieved the necessary level of conditioning, your focus can then shift to optimizing balance and symmetry and developing your physique to its fullest potential.

As a general rule, you should remain in the basic training phase until you've been training for at least a year. That said, some women are fast responders and can transition into the advanced program a bit more quickly. Only you can determine whether you're ready to take the next step. I again caution you about being overzealous, though. It's better to stick with the basic training phase until you are completely confident in your abilities. Pushing too fast too soon will shortchange your results and leave you overtrained.

What follows is the protocol for the basic training phase as well as a sample routine that illustrates how to put it all together.

COMPOSITION OF THE ROUTINE

As in the break-in phase, you again perform a total-body routine that works all major muscles in each session. Recall that total-body training allows frequent stimulation of your neuromuscular system. This remains important in this phase because you are still developing neuromotor patterns that allow the nervous system to activate muscles in the most efficient manner possible. A greater training frequency increases practice time on the lifts, facilitating coordinated exercise performance. These skills become invaluable in the more advanced stages of the program, in which you'll focus on honing the connection between mind and muscle to bring about optimal muscle development.

FREQUENCY

Continue to employ a three-days-per-week training schedule, working out on nonconsecutive days (e.g., Monday/Wednesday/Friday). This provides the requisite 48-hour rest needed for muscle protein synthesis to run its course as well as adequate time for overall neuromuscular recuperation.

Because you are increasing total training volume and intensity of effort, the demands on your neuromuscular system are substantially higher than they were in the break-in phase. Although the three-day structure of the routine generally provides sufficient recovery between workouts, both genetic and lifestyle factors influence individual response. The early stages in particular can overtax your recuperative capacity. Be in tune with your body. Don't hesitate to take an extra day off if needed. It's better to skip a workout than to run yourself down. Remember, muscle development occurs during rest, not when you're working out.

The same guidelines of the break-in phase apply to handling missed sessions in this phase. If you cannot work out on a given day, train on the following day and resume the alternate-day approach. For example, if you are on the Monday/Wednesday/Friday schedule and can't make the Monday session, then simply work out Tuesday/Thursday/Saturday instead. The following week you can resume your normal training schedule if desired. Again, do your best to get in three weekly workouts. Consistency is paramount for optimizing results.

EXERCISES

Given the total-body nature of the routine, this phase includes one exercise per muscle group. This keeps total intrasession training volume manageable so that you can channel all of your energies into each set. Moreover, weekly volume is maintained at a level conducive to recuperation, diminishing the likelihood of overtraining.

That said, exercise selection in this phase differs in several ways from that in the break-in phase.

For one, the basic training phase provides more exercise variety. The neuromuscular proficiency you established in the break-in phase transfers to an enhanced ability to perform a wide array of exercise variations. Employing an assortment of movements allows you to fully stimulate all the fibers of a given muscle, fostering complete development of your physique.

That said, there are diminishing returns to varying exercise selection. Changing exercises too frequently can cause you to spend more time learning new movement patterns rather than solidifying performance in exercises that will play a regular role in your rotation. There are no hard-and-fast rules here, but it's generally a good idea to maintain a core group of exercises (such as those employed in the break-in phase) as regular staples in your workout and then add variety around these movements.

This phase also incorporates single-joint exercises to complement the compound movements. Single-joint exercises help you target individual muscles or even aspects of a given muscle. However, this means that less overall muscle is stimulated during single-joint movements. Multijoint movements should therefore continue to form the basis of your exercise selection, comprising approximately two-thirds or more of the movements; the balance should be made up of single-joint exercises. Fortunately, single-joint movements generally involve less coordination than their multijoint counterparts. You should thus be able to get the hang of these exercises quite readily, facilitating more rapid muscle gains.

In addition, you'll now perform direct exercises for the arms, calves, and abs to enhance overall muscle development. By their nature, these muscle groups require the use of single-joint movements and are thus less taxing on the neuromuscular system. They therefore enhance development in the target muscles without compromising recovery. Note that these targeted exercises are included only in the moderate and light sessions; they are not suited for heavy lifting because of the large stresses they place on the joint, which increases the potential for injury.

SETS

The number of sets is based on the loading zone. For heavy loading sessions, perform four or five sets per exercise; for moderate loading sessions, perform three or four sets for exercises involving larger-muscle groups and two or three sets for those targeting smaller muscles. For light loading sessions, perform two or three sets per exercise. Note the increase in total training volume; at this point you should be able to handle the additional volume, particularly given that some of the work is in the form of single-joint movements, which are less taxing on the neuromuscular system. The multiset approach continues to provide ample practice time to fully ingrain neuromotor patterns while adding quality muscle to all the major muscle groups.

REPETITIONS

This phase introduces loading schemes. The loads used in these zones correspond to low-, medium-, and high-repetition ranges. Although you can gain muscle from training in pretty much any rep range, combining the loading zones produces a synergistic effect on muscle development, as discussed in chapter 2.

To acclimate your body to the loading zones, this phase employs a concept called daily undulating periodization (DUP), in which the number of rep ranges is manipulated over the course of each week. Session 1 is a heavy day of 3 to 5 reps per set; session 2 is a medium day of 8 to 12 reps per set; and session 3 is a light day of 15 to 25 reps per set. In this way you train through the spectrum of loading zones on a regular basis. One caveat: On heavy days, stick with multi-joint movements for the chest, shoulders, back, and hips and thighs. Moreover, when training the arms, calves, and abs on heavy days, perform 8 to 12 reps, because they require single-joint exercises that can overstress the joints when heavily loaded.

You'll no doubt notice big differences in the mind-set required for each loading zone. Heavy loading requires complete focus on moving the weights. You need to exert an all-out effort from the get-go. The goal is to move the weights as explosively as possible, even though actual lifting speed is rather slow. On the other hand, light load sets start off very easy but get quite uncomfortable as lactic acid begins to build up. By the end of the set, the acidosis will challenge your fortitude. You'll need to stay mentally strong and push past the discomfort to reap the desired rewards.

It is important to focus on developing a strong mind-to-muscle connection, in which you consciously engage the target muscles to carry out an exercise (see the sidebar Mind-to-Muscle Connection). This strategy is particularly applicable to training in the moderate- and high-rep ranges. Mastering this technique will take your physique to a whole new level.

REST INTERVALS

Rest intervals are adjusted according to the loading range in this phase. Because the primary goal of low-rep training is to increase absolute strength, more time is required between sets to allow sufficient recuperation before lifting heavy loads in the succeeding set. Alternatively, high-rep training benefits from short rest periods because they encourage the endurance-oriented adaptations associated with enhanced buffering capacity and nutrient delivery. Medium-rep training can benefit from a middle ground approach that provides sufficient intraset recovery so that mechanical tension is not significantly compromised while allowing for a time-efficient workout.

Adhere to the following rest guidelines in the basic training phase:

- When using low reps (3-5 per set), rest approximately 2 to 3 minutes between sets.
- When using moderate reps (8-12 per set), reduce the rest interval to approximately 90 to 120 seconds between sets.
- When using high reps (15-20 per set or more), limit your rest intervals further, resting approximately 30 to 60 seconds between sets.

INTENSITY OF EFFORT

You are amping up the intensity of effort in this phase. Sets are increasingly demanding, and you train regularly to muscle failure. This is necessary to fully stimulate the spectrum of muscle fibers. The only way to ensure consistent gains is to challenge your neuromuscular system beyond its present capacity. Pure and simple, this requires high levels of effort.

Mind-to-Muscle Connection

Contrary to what many believe, resistance training is not simply the act of lifting a weight from point A to point B. Because your mind plays an important role in the development of your physique, to get the most out of your efforts, you must harness its power. In fact, two women using identical exercise routines will achieve vastly different results based on their mental approaches to training.

What I'm talking about here is developing a mind-to-muscle connection—the melding of mind and muscle so that they become one. The mind-to-muscle connection entails visualizing the muscle you are training and feeling that muscle work throughout each repetition. Rather than thinking about where you feel a muscular stimulus, you must think about where you are *supposed* to feel the stimulus.

Establishing a mind-to-muscle connection is beneficial on two levels. First, it ensures that your target muscles perform the majority of the work during an exercise instead of allowing supporting muscles to dominate the lift. Now this doesn't mean that you isolate the intended muscles; complete muscular isolation is a near impossibility during traditional strength training. But you will maximize the work they perform, thus optimizing their development.

Second, it forces you to use proper form. When you are mentally locked in to a movement, your biomechanics tend to automatically fall into place. This not only improves exercise performance, but also reduces the possibility of a training-related injury.

Developing a strong mind-to-muscle connection requires consistent practice. From the moment you begin a set, your thoughts should be focused on the muscle you are training, with all outside distractions purged from your mind. The only thing that matters at this point is the task at hand: stimulating your target muscles to their fullest potential.

As you train, make a concerted effort to visualize your target muscles doing the work, without assistance from supporting muscles. When you reach the fully contracted concentric portion of the movement, consciously feel the squeeze in your target muscles. On the eccentric (i.e., negative) action, feel your target muscles lengthening as you return to the start position. Make this practice a ritual, and it soon will become a habit.

Don't be discouraged if developing a mental link takes longer with some muscles than with others. Generally speaking, connecting with the muscles of your arms and legs is easier than connecting with those of your torso. However, with dedication and patience, you'll be able to connect with all the muscles in your body, paving the way to better development.

You can enhance your mind-to-muscle connection through the use of a technique called guided imagery. With this technique, you visualize the way you want your muscles to appear and then imagine them taking this form as you are training. For instance, when working your triceps, envision yourself with firm, defined arms. As you perform a set of overhead triceps extensions, imagine your arms becoming tighter and harder. Make the image as vivid as possible. With each repetition, see yourself getting one step closer to achieving your goal. By tapping into the power of your subconscious mind, you can take your body to new heights, turning fantasy into reality.

You again use the reps-to-failure (RTF) scale to estimate effort for each set (see table 2.1 in chapter 2 for a description of the rating scale). Training intensity progressively increases over each set of each exercise, culminating in an all-out effort on the final set. Here is how it plays out:

- Set 1: Your level of effort on the initial set should correspond to an RTF of 2, equating to a very difficult intensity. Select a weight that allows you to achieve the target rep range with approximately two reps in reserve.

- Set 2: On the second set, your level of effort should correspond to an RTF of 1, equating to an extremely difficult intensity. Select a weight that allows you to achieve the target rep range with approximately one rep in reserve. The loads here are highly challenging because you are stopping just short of training to failure.
- Set 3: The final set should be taken to concentric muscular failure—the point at which you cannot complete another rep with good form (RTF of 0). Push yourself to the limit, giving everything you have to finish the set.

It's important to note the delicate balance between pushing yourself hard and overdoing it. Research shows that consistently training with high intensities of effort predisposes people to overtraining (Izquierdo et al., 2006). The protocol in this phase is designed to balance the level of effort expended so that you don't overtax your neuromuscular system. That said, individual differences in genetics and lifestyles ultimately dictate the response to training. This tends to be particularly pertinent during the beginning stages of transitioning to a more advanced stage because your body might not be as ready as your mind to endure the bump in intensity. If you feel overtaxed, pull back on the level of effort. Perhaps go to failure every other week, or even every third week. You can then increase the intensity gradually as your body adjusts to the demands of the routine.

Table 8.1 summarizes the basic training phase protocol. Sample routines are provided in table 8.2. These routines are intended to serve as a basic template for constructing your workouts. Modify exercises according to your needs and abilities.

Table 8.1   Summary of the Basic Training Phase

Training variable	Protocol
Sets	2-5 per exercise
Repetitions	3-25
Rest interval	30 sec to 3 min
Frequency	3 days a week

Table 8.2 Sample Basic Training Phase Routine

Monday (heavy)					
Exercise	Exercise photo	Sets	Repetitions	Rest interval	Page number
Dumbbell chest press		4 or 5	3-5	2-3 min	125
Dumbbell single-arm row		4 or 5	3-5	2-3 min	109
Military press		4 or 5	3-5	2-3 min	24
Barbell back squat		4 or 5	3-5	2-3 min	64
Barbell hip thrust		4 or 5	3-5	2-3 min	69
Barbell stiff-leg deadlift		4 or 5	3-5	2-3 min	82
Wednesday (moderate)					
Barbell incline press		3 or 4	8-12	90-120 sec	122
Neutral-grip lat pull-down		3 or 4	8-12	90-120 sec	106
Cable upright row		3 or 4	8-12	90-120 sec	27

(continued)

169

Table 8.2 Sample Basic Training Phase Routine *(continued)*

Exercise	Exercise photo	Sets	Repetitions	Rest interval	Page number
Wednesday (moderate)					
Dumbbell incline biceps curl		2 or 3	8-12	90-120 sec	37
Cable rope overhead triceps extension		2 or 3	8-12	90-120 sec	50
Leg press		3 or 4	8-12	90-120 sec	67
Machine seated leg curl		3 or 4	8-12	90-120 sec	91
Dumbbell standing calf raise		2 or 3	8-12	90-120 sec	96
Cable kneeling rope crunch		2 or 3	8-12	90-120 sec	140
Friday (light)					
Low cable fly		2 or 3	15-25	30-60 sec	130
Cable seated row		2 or 3	15-25	30-60 sec	112
Machine lateral raise		2 or 3	15-25	30-60 sec	30

Friday (light)					
Exercise	Exercise photo	Sets	Repetitions	Rest interval	Page number
Dumbbell hammer curl		2 or 3	15-25	30-60 sec	47
Cable triceps kickback		2 or 3	15-25	30-60 sec	54
Leg extension		2 or 3	15-25	30-60 sec	76
Cable glute back kick		2 or 3	15-25	30-60 sec	85
Machine seated calf raise		2 or 3	15-25	30-60 sec	98
Reverse crunch		2 or 3	15-25	30-60 sec	136

9

Advanced Body-Sculpting Phase

Kudos! The fact that you're about to start the advanced body-sculpting phase of the Strong and Sculpted program means that you're no longer a novice. You have at least a year of consistent resistance training experience under your belt, perhaps more. You've developed complete proficiency in exercise performance. You're able to push your body hard during each workout and have come back strong for the next one. Be proud of your accomplishment; you've surpassed the expertise of the majority of lifters.

You're now ready to take your physique to the next level.

The advanced body-sculpting phase focuses on bringing your physique into aesthetic proportion. To understand the process, let's again revisit the analogy of constructing a house. Recall that before building your dream house, you need to lay a solid foundation. Once the foundation is in place, you then erect the frame so that it has a structure. Only after these components are complete can you fill in the interior so the house truly takes shape.

From a body-sculpting standpoint, you've built the foundation and structure; now the real work begins!

The goal in this phase is to develop muscular symmetry in which each muscle flows into the next, creating balanced lines that complement one another. Although you can't change your God-given genes, you can change your shape. Body sculpting gives you the ability to alter your proportions in a manner that emphasizes your genetic strengths while concealing any weaknesses. For instance, let's say that you have a naturally blocky waist. For all practical purposes, there's nothing you can do to change this fact (unless perhaps you're one of those Hollywood starlets who opts to remove a rib or two). However, by selectively adding muscle to your middle deltoid and upper-back areas, you can increase your shoulder-to-waist differential, thereby creating the illusion of a smaller waist. Body sculpting is all about illusion. With proper knowledge and effort, you can mask your genetic limitations.

I won't sugarcoat things, though. The process isn't easy. It requires dedication and commitment. But assuming you have the desire, it's within your power to attain the physique you've always dreamed of having.

What follows is the protocol for the advanced body-sculpting phase as well as a sample routine that illustrates how to put it all together.

COMPOSITION OF THE ROUTINE

Previous phases of the Strong and Sculpted program employed a total-body routine that involved working all the major muscle groups in each training session. As discussed earlier, total-body routines are good for enhancing motor learning and developing basic strength. You have now achieved all of these attributes to the extent necessary for body sculpting.

It's now time to step things up another notch.

The advanced body-sculpting phase employs a split-body routine that involves multiple exercises performed for a limited number of muscle groups in a session. The primary advantage of a split routine is that it allows you to perform a higher volume of training while affording greater recovery between sessions. Recall that there is a clear dose–response relationship between training volume and muscle development: Up to a certain point, higher volumes translate into better results. Sure, it's possible to increase volume in a total-body routine by extending the length of the training session. But the downside of such an approach is that your energy levels dissipate over the course of the training bout, compromising your ability to sustain training intensity. With split routines, sessions can be kept relatively brief, allowing you to maintain intensity throughout the bout. Moreover, split routines can increase metabolic stress by prolonging the training stimulus within a given muscle group, thereby heightening the acute factors responsible for muscle development. The result is an enhanced capacity for shaping your muscles to their ultimate potential.

FREQUENCY

In this phase, workout frequency is increased from three to four days a week. An upper and lower split-body routine is performed in a two-on and one-off, two-on and two-off fashion. Simply stated, this means that you work out two days in a row, take a day off, work out two days in a row, and then take two days off. A typical training scheme in this format involves training Monday, Tuesday, Thursday, and Friday, although other permutations are fine as well (e.g., Tuesday, Wednesday, Saturday, and Sunday). Alternatively, you can employ a two-on and one-off, one-on and one-off, and one-on and one-off schedule (e.g., training Monday, Tuesday, Thursday, and Saturday). To optimize recovery, it's generally best to avoid training more than two days in a row on this schedule. However, if you run into issues during a given week, a three-on and two-off, one-on and one-off schedule is a viable, albeit less desirable, option. The bottom line is that as long as you get in the four training days per week and provide sufficient recovery, all is good.

To quote the Nike slogan: Just do it!

EXERCISES

In this phase you perform two or three exercises per muscle group per session (instead of a single exercise as in previous phases). You should now be more cognizant of choosing exercises that are complementary from a muscle development standpoint. One of the biggest training mistakes I see is haphazardly stringing together a series of exercises without consideration of how they interact with each other. The effect is a hodgepodge of movements with little cohesion. Ultimately, if you want to rise above the ordinary and maximize your genetic potential, a more scientific approach is in order. Fortunately, the Strong and Sculpted program makes it easy to accomplish this task.

The exercises described in chapters 3 through 5 are segmented into categories based on movement patterns for each muscle group. Following are guidelines for combining these categories for optimal effect. Simply follow the guidelines as outlined, and you'll have a perfect workout every time. Guaranteed!

• *Shoulders*: For moderate and light sessions, choose one multijoint shoulder exercise (shoulder category 1) and one single-joint shoulder exercise (shoulder categories 2 and 3) for each workout. With respect to the single-joint movement, make sure to vary these exercises by planes of movement. Specifically, alternate between a frontal plane movement targeting the middle delts (shoulder category 2) and a transverse plane movement targeting the rear delts (shoulder category 3) from workout to workout. For heavy sessions, choose one multijoint shoulder exercise (shoulder category 1); avoid single-joint movements during these sessions because of the high stresses they place on the joints.

• *Back*: For moderate and light sessions, choose one multijoint pull-down or pull-up exercise (back category 1) and one multijoint row exercise (back category 2) each workout. If desired, you can substitute a single-joint exercise (back category 3) for either the pull-down or pull-up or the row movement, but no more than every other workout. For heavy sessions, choose one multijoint pull-down or pull-up exercise (back category 1) and one multijoint row exercise (back category 2); avoid single-joint movements during these sessions because of the high stresses they put on the joints.

• *Chest*: For moderate and light sessions, choose one multijoint chest exercise (chest categories 1 and 2) and one single-joint exercise (chest categories 3 and 4) for each workout. The multijoint exercise should vary between an upper-chest exercise (chest category 1) and a midchest exercise (chest category 2). Similarly, the single-joint exercise should vary between an upper-chest exercise (chest category 3) and a midchest exercise (chest category 4). For heavy sessions, choose one multijoint shoulder exercise (chest categories 1 and 2); avoid single-joint movements during these sessions because of the high stresses they put on the joints.

• *Elbow flexors*: For moderate and light sessions, choose one exercise that is carried out with your arms at your sides or behind your body (elbow flexor category 1) and one that is carried out with your arms in front of your body or raised to your sides (elbow flexor category 2). Every other workout, substitute an exercise carried out with your hands either pronated or in a neutral position (elbow flexor category 3). Exercises directly targeting the elbow flexors should be avoided during heavy sessions because of the high stresses they place on the joints.

• *Elbow extensors*: For moderate and light sessions, choose one exercise that is carried out with your arms overhead (elbow extensor category 1) and one that's carried out with your arms at your sides (elbow extensor category 2). Every other workout, substitute an exercise with your arms midway between overhead and at your sides (elbow extensor category 3). Exercises directly targeting the elbow extensors should be avoided during heavy sessions because of the high stresses they place on the joints.

• *Frontal thighs and hips*: For moderate and light sessions, choose one multijoint bilateral exercise (frontal thigh and hip category 1), one multijoint unilateral exercise (frontal thigh and hip category 2), and one single-joint exercise (frontal thigh and hip category 3) each workout. Single-joint exercises should be avoided during heavy sessions because of the high stresses they place on the joints.

• *Posterior thighs and hips*: For moderate and light sessions, choose one exercise that targets the glutes and hamstrings through hip extension (posterior thigh and hip category 1) and one exercise that targets the hamstrings through knee flexion (posterior thigh and hip category 2). For heavy sessions, choose two exercises targeting the hamstrings through hip extension (posterior thigh and hip category 1).

• *Calves*: For moderate and light sessions, choose one straight-leg exercise (calf category 1) and one bent-leg exercise (calf category 2). Exercises directly targeting the calves should be avoided during heavy sessions because of the high stresses they place on the joints.

• *Abdominals*: For moderate and light sessions, choose one exercise involving spinal flexion (abdominal category 1) and one exercise involving rotation or lateral flexion (abdominal category 2). Every other workout, substitute an exercise that statically challenges the abdominals (abdominal category 3) for either a category 1 or category 2 movement. Exercises directly targeting the abs should be avoided during heavy sessions because of the high stresses they place on the joints.

SETS

As in the basic training phase, the number of sets in this phase is based on the loading zone employed. For heavy loading sessions, perform five or six sets for the frontal thigh and hip exercises and four or five sets per exercise for the posterior thighs and hips. For moderate loading sessions, perform three or four sets for exercises involving larger-muscle groups and two or three sets for those targeting smaller muscles. For light loading sessions, perform two or three sets per exercise. However, because you're now using two or three exercises for each muscle group, you'll perform a total of six to nine sets for that muscle per workout (as opposed to previous phases in which you performed only three sets per muscle group per workout). Initially, this increase in intrasession training volume promotes significant muscular fatigue. Expect to have reduced energy levels for several weeks until your body adapts to this additional workload. Within a short time, though, you will have adjusted to these demands, and your exercise tolerance will have improved dramatically.

REPETITIONS

As in the basic training phase, the advanced body-sculpting phase incorporates a daily undulating periodization (DUP) scheme in which the repetitions are varied from workout to workout. To accommodate the split-body nature of this phase, the DUP is modified so that you train the full spectrum of repetition ranges every 10 days or so (as opposed to every week in the previous phases). Specifically, heavy (3-5 reps), moderate (8-12 reps), and light (15-25 reps) workouts are split up so that they are worked over two sessions. In the two-on and one-off, two-on and two-off schedule, this means Monday and Tuesday are heavy-load days, Thursday and Friday are moderate-load days, and the following Monday and Tuesday are light-load days. The cycle then repeats with heavy-load training commencing on the subsequent Thursday.

REST INTERVALS

As in the basic training phase, rest intervals are adjusted according to the loading range. Adhere to the following guidelines:

- When using low reps (3-5 per set), take approximately two- to three-minute rests between sets.
- When using moderate reps (8-12 per set), reduce the rest interval so that you rest approximately 90 to 120 seconds between sets.
- When using high reps (15-20 per set or more), limit rest intervals further, resting approximately 30 to 60 seconds or less between sets.

INTENSITY OF EFFORT

You will again use the reps-to-failure (RTF) scale to estimate effort for each set (see table 2.1 in chapter 2 for a description of the rating scale). The level of effort is further increased here, so that the initial sets are all highly challenging. The final set is performed in an all-out fashion. Here is how it plays out:

- Sets 1 and 2: Your level of effort on the first two sets should correspond to an RTF of 1, equating to an extremely difficult intensity. This entails selecting a weight that allows you to achieve the target rep range with approximately one rep in reserve. The sets here are highly challenging because you are stopping just short of training to failure.
- Set 3: The final set should be carried out to the point of concentric muscular failure—the point at which you cannot complete another rep with good form. This corresponds to an RTF of 0. You're going all out here, leaving nothing in reserve after squeezing out the last rep.

DELOADS

In the advanced body-sculpting phase, you are working probably harder than you've ever worked before. Although such intensity is necessary to optimize results, it ultimately takes a toll on your body. As discussed in chapter 2, consistently pushing yourself to the max will ultimately lead to an overtrained state. This not only has negative effects on your health status, but also can impair muscle development.

To ensure that your efforts do not devolve into overtraining, this phase of the program incorporates regular deload cycles in which both the volume and intensity of training are systematically reduced for a short period of time, generally a full week. The deload periods are designed to restore the function of your muscles and joints and allow your neuromuscular system to recover from the extreme demands of hard training. After the deload, you should feel refreshed and rejuvenated, stoked to push yourself even harder than before.

As a general rule, deloads should be instituted every four to six weeks or so. However, the frequency is highly individual and depends on a diverse array of factors including genetics, training experience, nutritional status, stress, sleep, and other lifestyle factors. Find a frequency that works best for you. I recommend starting with monthly deloads (i.e., three weeks of hard training followed by a one-week deload). Then adjust the frequency based on your response. Just make sure that you take an objective approach. Don't let your quest for attaining a great physique blind you to your physical state. If you're feeling run down, take a deload week.

During your deload cycles, train two days per week, allowing 72 hours between sessions (e.g., Monday and Thursday). Use a total-body routine in which you work all the major muscle groups in each session. Perform two or three sets of one exercise per muscle group targeting approximately 15-20 reps per set, with a rest interval of about two minutes between sets. Sets should not be overly challenging. Aim for an RTF of 3 or so (i.e., the target rep range is achieved with about three reps left in reserve). If you are struggling on the last few reps, lighten the weight!

SPECIAL TRAINING TECHNIQUE

To enhance the training effect, the advanced body-sculpting phase introduces the judicious use of a technique called supersets. A superset is two exercises carried out in succession without rest. Although supersets can be performed in a variety of ways, I recommend using reciprocal supersets (i.e., alternating exercises that share an agonist–antagonist relationship). Examples of reciprocal supersets are biceps/triceps, back/chest, and quadriceps/hamstrings.

Reciprocal supersets have an inherent advantage over other superset variations: They cause little if any reduction in your strength. In fact, studies indicate that by contracting an antagonist muscle, you can actually increase force output during subsequent contractions of the agonist (Carregaro et al., 2013). This is presumably the result of reduced antagonist inhibition and possibly stored elastic energy in the muscle–tendon complex. And as you know by now, greater muscle tension generated by the agonist leads to better muscular development, particularly in the presence of high amounts of metabolic stress.

Here's how it should play out: Perform a set of the first exercise, proceed directly to the second exercise as quickly as possible, rest for the prescribed amount of time, and then repeat for two additional supersets. Then move on to the next agonist–antagonist pairing, and so on until you have completed all paired sets. Ideally, it's best to set up exercise stations in advance so that you can move quickly between exercises. You can choose to superset as many or as few of the paired muscle groups as you like, but limit the use of this technique to moderate and light sessions.

Table 9.1 summarizes the advanced body-sculpting phase protocol. Sample routines are provided in table 9.2. These routines are intended to serve as a basic template for constructing your workouts. Modify exercises according to your needs and abilities.

Table 9.1 Summary of the Advanced Body-Sculpting Phase

	Body region	Sets	Repetitions	Rest interval
Day 1 (heavy)	Lower	4-6	3-5	2-3 min
Day 2 (heavy)	Upper	5-6	3-5	2-3 min
Day 1 (moderate)	Lower and abs	2-4	8-12	90-120 sec
Day 2 (moderate)	Upper	2-4	8-12	90-120 sec
Day 1 (light)	Lower and abs	2-3	15-25	30-60 sec
Day 2 (light)	Upper	2-3	15-25	30-60 sec

Table 9.2 Sample Advanced Body-Sculpting Phase Routine

WEEK 1					
Monday (heavy lower)					
Exercise	Exercise photo	Sets	Repetitions	Rest interval	Page number
Goblet squat		5 or 6	3-5	2-3 min	66
Deadlift		5 or 6	3-5	2-3 min	63
Leg press		5 or 6	3-5	2-3 min	67
Barbell glute bridge		4 or 5	3-5	2-3 min	83
Dumbbell stiff-leg deadlift		4 or 5	3-5	2-3 min	82

(continued)

Table 9.2 Sample Advanced Body-Sculpting Phase Routine *(continued)*

WEEK 1

Tuesday (heavy upper)

Exercise	Exercise photo	Sets	Repetitions	Rest interval	Page number
Barbell chest press		5 or 6	3-5	2-3 min	127
Pull-up		5 or 6	3-5	2-3 min	104
Machine shoulder press		5 or 6	3-5	2-3 min	26
Barbell reverse bent row		5 or 6	3-5	2-3 min	111

Thursday (moderate lower and abs)

Barbell front squat		3 or 4	8-12	90-120 sec	65
Bulgarian split squat		3 or 4	8-12	90-120 sec	68
Barbell hip thrust		3 or 4	8-12	90-120 sec	84
Hyperextension		3 or 4	8-12	90-120 sec	87
Lying leg curl		2 or 3	8-12	90-120 sec	89

Thursday (moderate lower and abs)

Exercise	Exercise photo	Sets	Repetitions	Rest interval	Page number
Machine standing calf raise		2 or 3	8-12	90-120 sec	95
Barbell kneeling rollout		2 or 3	8-12	90-120 sec	138
Cable side bend		2 or 3	8-12	90-120 sec	144

Friday (moderate upper)

Exercise	Exercise photo	Sets	Repetitions	Rest interval	Page number
Machine incline press		3 or 4	8-12	90-120 sec	123
Flat dumbbell fly		3 or 4	8-12	90-120 sec	131
Lat pull-down		3 or 4	8-12	90-120 sec	105
Cable wide-grip seated row		3 or 4	8-12	90-120 sec	113
Dumbbell shoulder press		3 or 4	8-12	90-120 sec	23

(continued)

Table 9.2 Sample Advanced Body-Sculpting Phase Routine *(continued)*

WEEK 1					
Friday (moderate upper)					
Exercise	**Exercise photo**	**Sets**	**Repetitions**	**Rest interval**	**Page number**
Cable lateral raise		3 or 4	8-12	90-120 sec	29
Barbell drag curl		2 or 3	8-12	90-120 sec	38
Dumbbell prone incline curl		2 or 3	8-12	90-120 sec	43
Machine overhead triceps extension		2 or 3	8-12	90-120 sec	52
Triceps dip		2 or 3	8-12	90-120 sec	55
WEEK 2					
Monday (light lower and abs)					
Dumbbell reverse lunge		2 or 3	15-25	30-60 sec	70
Single-leg extension		2 or 3	15-25	30-60 sec	77
Cable standing abduction		2 or 3	15-25	30-60 sec	88
Machine seated leg curl		2 or 3	15-25	30-60 sec	91

Monday (light lower and abs)

Exercise	Exercise photo	Sets	Repetitions	Rest interval	Page number
Reverse hyperextension		2 or 3	15-25	30-60 sec	86
Machine seated calf raise		2 or 3	15-25	30-60 sec	98
Toe press		2 or 3	15-25	30-60 sec	94
Reverse crunch		2 or 3	15-25	30-60 sec	136
Side bridge		2 or 3	15-25	30-60 sec	148
Tuesday (light upper)					
Dumbbell decline press		2 or 3	15-25	30-60 sec	124
Pec deck fly		2 or 3	15-25	30-60 sec	133
Cross cable pull-down		2 or 3	15-25	30-60 sec	108
Cable single-arm standing low row		2 or 3	15-25	30-60 sec	116

(continued)

Table 9.2 Sample Advanced Body-Sculpting Phase Routine *(continued)*

WEEK 2

Tuesday (light upper)

Exercise	Exercise photo	Sets	Repetitions	Rest interval	Page number
Dumbbell upright row		2 or 3	15-25	30-60 sec	25
Cable reverse fly		2 or 3	15-25	30-60 sec	32
Cable curl		2 or 3	15-25	30-60 sec	40
Barbell reverse curl		2 or 3	15-25	30-60 sec	48
Dumbbell overhead triceps extension		2 or 3	15-25	30-60 sec	51
Skull crusher		2 or 3	15-25	30-60 sec	57

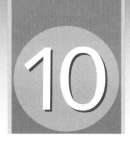

Peak Physique Phase

If you've followed the program as outlined to this point, you'll have developed an impressive physique. In fact, you should be able to reach upwards of 95 percent of your genetic potential from adhering to the principles laid out in the previous phases of the program. If you're satisfied with the results you've achieved so far, great! It's perfectly fine to continue along the same path. You'll look and feel great for as long as you put in the required effort. But if you want to take your physique to its ultimate potential, a more demanding program is in order.

Enter the peak physique phase of the Strong and Sculpted program.

The peak physique phase is an intensive three-week routine that requires an increased commitment of time and effort over previous phases. You'll be pushed to your physical limits. Your resolve will be consistently challenged. But if you aspire to achieve your best body ever, the results will be well worth it.

Maximal muscle development is accomplished by bringing about a phenomenon called functional overreaching. Think of it as going to the edge of the overtraining cliff without falling off. The impelling force here is an increase in training volume. Recall that volume is a primary driver of muscular adaptations; that is, higher volumes lead to greater muscle development—at least to a point.

The problem is that the body's capacity to recover from repeated bouts of intense, high-volume exercise is limited. Consistently training with high volumes is bound to exceed your capacity to recover and thus have a detrimental effect on results. Fortunately, this doesn't pose an issue over short periods of time. In fact, when the body is subjected to a brief high-volume training cycle, it supercompensates by remodeling muscle tissue above and beyond what can be achieved otherwise. But push the envelope too far, and you're bound to wind up overtrained.

Thus, manipulating volume for maximal muscular development becomes a balancing act in which higher-volume periods are selectively interspersed with lower-volume periods. In essence, you must straddle the line between pushing yourself to the edge of the cliff and going too far. That's why the peak physique phase is followed by an active recovery period in which you abstain from any intense training. During this period the full effects of supercompensation manifest, which is why allowing adequate recuperation is essential to realizing optimal results.

As a general rule, the peak physique phase should be performed no more than every three months or so to avoid an overtrained state. Once you have completed the phase, return to the advanced body-sculpting phase as your go-to long-term training plan.

Moreover, keep in mind that people respond differently to the stresses of exercise. Although I've structured this phase to provide functional overreaching without leaving you overtrained, it's imperative that you stay in tune with your body. Don't hesitate to alter aspects of the routine based on how you feel. Alterations can be made on a daily or weekly basis by reducing volume, intensity, or a combination of the two. Remember, customizing your training to your needs and abilities is the key to optimizing results.

What follows is the protocol for the peak physique phase as well as a sample routine that illustrates how to put it all together.

COMPOSITION OF THE ROUTINE

The peak physique phase employs a split-body routine in which multiple exercises are performed for a limited number of muscle groups each session. As noted in chapter 9, split-body routines allow you to perform a higher volume of training while affording greater recovery between sessions. Because volume is a primary driver of muscle development, you'll be upping the number of weekly sets per muscle group to tax your body to its limits.

Unlike the advanced body-sculpting phase, which employed a two-day split routine, in this phase you perform a three-day split in which day 1 addresses the back, chest, and abs; day 2 addresses the lower body; and day 3 addresses the shoulders and arms. Splitting the routine so that fewer muscle groups are trained allows you to perform more exercises per muscle group, and thus facilitates your ability to target specific portions of each muscle. The additional sets per muscle group during each workout also increase the extent of metabolic buildup in the working muscles, providing a greater hypothetical stimulus for development.

FREQUENCY

Workout frequency in this phase is increased to six days a week, employing a three-on and one-off schedule. In simple terms, you'll work out three days in a row, take a day off, and then repeat the process throughout the training block. The higher training frequency bumps up volume without increasing the duration of your workouts. This allows you to go all out each session, leaving nothing in reserve.

You will likely begin to experience fatigue over the course of this training phase. Usually, the first week goes OK. You're probably fueled by adrenaline, amped from the excitement and anticipation of maximizing results. But by the second or third week, the demands of the program will probably begin to take a toll, both physically and mentally. You'll need to draw on your inner strength to maintain training focus. Remember, the objective here is to promote overreaching. This entails giving 100 percent in every workout; if you slack off, results inevitably suffer.

EXERCISES

In this phase you perform two to four exercises per muscle group per session. Exercise selection here is paramount. Your focus should be on developing optimal symmetry between muscles. Each muscle should be in balance with its opposing muscle, as well as in the context of your overall physique. Genetics dictate that certain muscles will respond extremely well to training, whereas others will lag. You'll therefore need to be objectively critical of your physique.

It's all too common for people to focus on the muscles they care about most and ignore the others. Don't fall into this trap. A body should be in balance so that no one muscle stands out over another. To this end, you should differentiate the muscle groups that are your strong points from those that are weaknesses, and prioritize your training accordingly. Adjust the volume so that lagging muscles get more work at the expense of the muscles that respond easily to training. Moreover, train the laggards first in your workout when you are fresh to ensure maximal effort.

To develop your body to its fullest, you need to be sure that you work the muscles from all possible angles in all planes of movement. Fortunately, this program makes the task easy to accomplish. For best results, follow these fool-proof guidelines:

- *Shoulders*: Choose one multijoint shoulder exercise (shoulder category 1) and two single-joint shoulder exercises (shoulder categories 2 and 3) for each workout. With respect to the single-joint movements, choose one frontal plane movement targeting the middle delts (shoulder category 2) and one transverse plane movement targeting the rear delts (shoulder category 3) to ensure the complete development of all three deltoid heads.

- *Back*: Choose one multijoint pull-down or pull-up exercise (back category 1), one multijoint row exercise (back category 2), and one single-joint exercise (back category 3) for each workout. Also, vary between close-grip and wide-grip variations in the multijoint movements.

- *Chest*: Choose two multijoint chest exercises (chest categories 1 and 2) and one single-joint exercise (chest categories 3 and 4) for each workout. With respect to the multijoint exercises, workouts should include both an upper-chest exercise (chest category 1) and a midchest exercise (chest category 2). The single-joint exercise should rotate between an upper-chest exercise (chest category 3) and a midchest exercise (chest category 4) from one workout to the next.

- *Elbow flexors*: Choose one exercise that is carried out with your arms at your sides or behind your body (elbow flexor category 1), one exercise that is carried out with your arms in front of your body or raised to your sides (elbow flexor category 2), and one exercise carried out with your hands either pronated or in a neutral position (elbow flexor category 3). Alternatively, choose two of these positions and rotate in the third as desired.

- *Elbow extensors*: Choose one exercise that is carried out with your arms overhead (elbow extensor category 1), one exercise that is carried out with your arms at your sides (elbow extensor category 2), and one exercise with your arms midway between overhead and at your sides (elbow extensor category 3). Alternatively, choose two of these positions and rotate in the third as desired.

- *Frontal thighs and hips*: Choose one multijoint bilateral exercise (frontal thigh and hip category 1), one multijoint unilateral exercise (frontal thigh and hip category 2), and one single-joint exercise (frontal thigh and hip category 3) for each workout.

- *Posterior thighs and hips*: Choose one exercise that targets the glutes and hamstrings through hip extension (posterior thigh and hip category 1) and one exercise that targets the hamstrings through knee flexion (posterior thigh and hip category 2).

• *Calves*: Choose one straight-leg exercise (calf category 1) and one bent-leg exercise (calf category 2).

• *Abdominals*: Choose one exercise involving spinal flexion (abdominal category 1) and one exercise involving rotation or lateral flexion (abdominal category 2). Every other workout, substitute an exercise that statically challenges the abdominals (abdominal category 3) for either a category 1 or a category 2 movement.

SETS

In this phase you perform 2 to 4 sets for each exercise, equating to 6 to 12 sets per muscle group per session. Larger muscles such as those in the back, chest, and thighs receive higher volumes, whereas the muscles of the arms and lower legs receive lower volumes given their smaller size and the fact that they function as secondary muscle movers in many mulitjoint exercises. Because each muscle group is worked twice per week, your total weekly volume is 16 to 24 sets per muscle group.

The increased volume brings about additional fatigue when training a given muscle. Metabolic buildup increases significantly with each successive set, causing you to really feel the burn. To an extent, your body will adapt to these demands by enhancing buffering capacity. However, you'll still need to push past the discomfort to reap the full rewards of the program. This is particularly important at the very advanced levels of training because the body needs greater and greater challenges to disturb homeostasis in a manner that promotes adaptation.

REPETITIONS

In the peak physique phase, you carry out sets in the 6- to 12-rep range. A step-loading approach is employed whereby you progressively increase the loads within the target rep range. This creates a wavelike loading pattern that allows you to train through the spectrum of medium loads in a concentrated fashion. Here's how it plays out in practice:

• Week 1: Target a loading zone of 10 to 12 reps per set.

• Week 2: Target a loading zone of 8 to 10 reps per set.

• Week 3: Target a loading zone of 6 to 8 reps per set.

REST INTERVALS

Rest intervals are consistent with previous recommendations for medium-load training—that is, approximately 90 to 120 seconds between sets. This provides sufficient intraset recovery so that mechanical tension is not significantly compromised while maintaining high amounts of intramuscular metabolic stress. The upshot is broad-based stimulation of the spectrum of muscle fibers while at the same time generating a good pump—a combination ideal for maximizing muscle development.

INTENSITY OF EFFORT

To promote functional overreaching, the level of effort in this phase is extremely high. Here's how things should play out using the reps-to-failure (RTF) scale from table 2.1 in chapter 2 to estimate effort:

- Weeks 1 and 2: Your level of effort on all sets except the final one should correspond to a 1 on the RTF scale. From a practical standpoint, this equates to selecting a weight that allows you to achieve the target rep range with just 1 additional rep in reserve. The final set should be performed to momentary muscular failure, leaving nothing in the tank.

- Week 3: All sets should be taken to the point of momentary muscular failure at which performance of another rep is not possible. It's not easy to push yourself to the limit throughout every workout, so stay focused on the ultimate goal of attaining your peak physique. And remember that it'll be over within a week's time; afterward, you will reap the rewards of your labor!

SPECIAL TRAINING TECHNIQUE

The peak physique phase incorporates drop sets (a.k.a. strip sets or descending sets). A drop set involves training to the point of failure on a given set, and then decreasing the load by about 25 percent and immediately performing as many additional reps as possible with the reduced weight. This technique enhances muscle fiber fatigue and metabolic stress. You should aim to strip off the weights as quickly as possible; resting more than a few seconds between drop sets diminishes the effects of the technique. If you're really feeling ambitious, you can perform multiple drops in the same set to elicit even greater fatigue and stress.

Perform drop sets on the final set of each exercise only. This is an advanced training technique that really taxes your recuperative abilities. Using the technique too frequently will ultimately lead to overtraining and psychological burnout.

ACTIVE RECOVERY

By the end of week 3, you should have pushed yourself to the limits of functional overreaching. It's therefore important to take a week or two off from training at this point to allow for optimal restoration of your body's resources and avoid the potential for overtraining. This doesn't mean that you should be a slug, hanging out on the couch all day watching TV. To the contrary, consider your time off as an active recovery phase in which you take part in light physical activities of your liking.

As a general rule, activities during your active recovery should be aerobic and performed at an intensity below your lactate threshold for 30 to 40 minutes on most days of the week. Exercise modalities should preferably address both upper- and lower-body musculature (e.g., elliptical trainers, cross-country ski trainers, jumping jacks) to enhance blood flow throughout your body. Sporting activities such as tennis and golf (no golf cart!) are fine as well. However, avoid resistance training during this time.

Remember, the active recovery period is a time for your body to catch up to the intense stresses placed on it during the training protocol by supercompensating with increased muscle development. Although it may be tempting to get right back in the gym and hit the weights, you mustn't shortchange this process. Doing so will serve only to impair the remodeling of muscle tissue and interfere with results. Worse, it can leave you overtrained, thereby setting back your progress for an extended period of time.

Table 10.1 summarizes the peak physique phase protocol. Sample routines are provided in table 10.2. These routines are intended to serve as a basic template for constructing your workouts. Modify exercises according to your needs and abilities.

Table 10.1   Summary of the Peak Physique Phase

	Body region	Sets	Repetitions	Rest interval
Monday	Back, chest, abs	3 or 4	6-12	90-120 sec
Tuesday	Lower body	3 or 4	6-12	90-120 sec
Wednesday	Shoulders, arms	2-4	6-12	90-120 sec
Thursday	Off	N/A	N/A	N/A
Friday	Back, chest, abs	3 or 4	6-12	90-120 sec
Saturday	Lower body	3 or 4	6-12	90-120 sec
Sunday	Shoulders, arms	2-4	6-12	90-120 sec

Table 10.2 Sample Peak Physique Phase Routine

	WEEK 1				
	Monday/Friday (back, chest, abs)				
Exercise	Exercise photo	Sets	Repetitions	Rest interval	Page number
Reverse-grip lat pull-down		4	10-12	90-120 sec	107
Machine seated row		4	10-12	90-120 sec	114
Dumbbell pullover		3	10-12	90-120 sec	118
Dumbbell incline press		4	10-12	90-120 sec	121
Barbell decline press		3	10-12	90-120 sec	126
Mid cable fly		3	10-12	90-120 sec	132
Hanging knee raise		3	10-12	90-120 sec	137
Bicycle crunch		3	10-12	90-120 sec	142

(continued)

Table 10.2 Sample Peak Physique Phase Routine *(continued)*

WEEK 1

Tuesday/Saturday (lower body)

Exercise	Exercise photo	Sets	Repetitions	Rest interval	Page number
Barbell front squat		4	10-12	90-120 sec	65
Dumbbell side lunge		4	10-12	90-120 sec	71
Sissy squat		3	10-12	90-120 sec	78
Good morning		4	10-12	90-120 sec	80
Stability ball leg curl		4	10-12	90-120 sec	92
Dumbbell single-leg standing calf raise		4	10-12	90-120 sec	97
Machine seated calf raise		3	10-12	90-120 sec	98

Wednesday/Sunday (shoulders, arms)

Exercise	Exercise photo	Sets	Repetitions	Rest interval	Page number
Dumbbell shoulder press		4	10-12	90-120 sec	23
Cable lateral raise		3	10-12	90-120 sec	29

Wednesday/Sunday (shoulders, arms)

Exercise	Exercise photo	Sets	Repetitions	Rest interval	Page number
Machine rear deltoid fly		3	10-12	90-120 sec	34
Dumbbell biceps curl		3	10-12	90-120 sec	36
Cable rope hammer curl		3	10-12	90-120 sec	46
Cable rope overhead triceps extension		3	10-12	90-120 sec	50
Dumbbell triceps kickback		2	10-12	90-120 sec	56
Close-grip bench press		2	10-12	90-120 sec	59

WEEK 2

Monday/Friday (back, chest, abs)

Lat pull-down		4	8-10	90-120 sec	105
T-bar row		4	8-10	90-120 sec	110

(continued)

Table 10.2 Sample Peak Physique Phase Routine *(continued)*

WEEK 2					
Monday/Friday (back, chest, abs)					
Exercise	**Exercise photo**	**Sets**	**Repetitions**	**Rest interval**	**Page number**
Cable straight-arm pull-down		3	8-10	90-120 sec	119
Machine incline press		4	8-10	90-120 sec	123
Dumbbell decline press		3	8-10	90-120 sec	124
Low cable fly		3	8-10	90-120 sec	130
Crunch		3	8-10	90-120 sec	135
Stability ball side crunch		3	8-10	90-120 sec	146
Tuesday/Saturday (lower body)					
Leg press		4	8-10	90-120 sec	67
Dumbbell step-up		4	8-10	90-120 sec	72
Single-leg extension		3	8-10	90-120 sec	77

WEEK 2

Tuesday/Saturday (lower body)

Exercise	Exercise photo	Sets	Repetitions	Rest interval	Page number
Barbell hip thrust		4	8-10	90-120 sec	84
Machine kneeling leg curl		4	8-10	90-120 sec	90
Toe press		3	8-10	90-120 sec	94
Machine single-leg seated calf raise		3	8-10	90-120 sec	99

Wednesday/Sunday (shoulders, arms)

Exercise	Exercise photo	Sets	Repetitions	Rest interval	Page number
Cable upright row		4	8-10	90-120 sec	27
Dumbbell lateral raise		4	8-10	90-120 sec	28
Cable kneeling bent reverse fly		3	8-10	90-120 sec	33
Barbell curl		2	8-10	90-120 sec	39
Concentration curl		2	8-10	90-120 sec	42

(continued)

Table 10.2 Sample Peak Physique Phase Routine *(continued)*

WEEK 2					
Wednesday/Sunday (shoulders, arms)					
Exercise	**Exercise photo**	**Sets**	**Repetitions**	**Rest interval**	**Page number**
Dumbbell hammer curl		2	8-10	90-120 sec	47
Machine overhead triceps extension		3	8-10	90-120 sec	52
Dumbbell lying triceps extension		3	8-10	90-120 sec	58
WEEK 3					
Monday/Friday (back, chest, abs)					
Chin-up		4	6-8	90-120 sec	103
Machine wide-grip seated row		4	6-8	90-120 sec	115
Dumbbell pullover		3	6-8	90-120 sec	118
Barbell incline press		4	6-8	90-120 sec	122
Machine chest press		3	6-8	90-120 sec	128

WEEK 3

Monday/Friday (back, chest, abs)

Exercise	Exercise photo	Sets	Repetitions	Rest interval	Page number
Dumbbell incline fly		3	6-8	90-120 sec	129
Cable kneeling rope crunch		3	6-8	90-120 sec	140
Antirotation press		3	6-8	90-120 sec	149

Tuesday/Saturday (lower body)

Exercise	Exercise photo	Sets	Repetitions	Rest interval	Page number
Barbell back squat		4	6-8	90-120 sec	64
Dumbbell lunge		4	6-8	90-120 sec	69
Leg extension		3	6-8	90-120 sec	76
Barbell stiff-leg deadlift		4	6-8	90-120 sec	81
Machine seated leg curl		3	6-8	90-120 sec	91
Machine standing calf raise		3	6-8	90-120 sec	95

(continued)

Table 10.2 Sample Peak Physique Phase Routine *(continued)*

WEEK 3					
Tuesday/Saturday (lower body)					
Exercise	**Exercise photo**	**Sets**	**Repetitions**	**Rest interval**	**Page number**
Machine seated calf raise		3	6-8	90-120 sec	98
Wednesday/Sunday (shoulders, arms)					
Military press		3	6-8	90-120 sec	24
Machine lateral raise		4	6-8	90-120 sec	30
Dumbbell seated bent reverse fly		3	6-8	90-120 sec	31
Dumbbell incline biceps curl		3	6-8	90-120 sec	37
High-pulley cable curl		3	6-8	90-120 sec	44
Dumbbell overhead triceps extension		3	6-8	90-120 sec	51
Cable triceps press-down		2	6-8	90-120 sec	53
Skull crusher		2	6-8	90-120 sec	57
WEEK 4 (ACTIVE RECOVERY): 1 WEEK OF LIGHT RECREATIONAL ACTIVITY ONLY					

Cardio Connection

Most women consider aerobic exercise (a.k.a. cardio, or cardiorespiratory exercise) essential in their quest to get lean. And without question, performing cardio can help to reduce body fat. If nothing else, energy expenditure is increased during physical activity, and if you burn more calories than you consume, you'll lose weight. There are two basic factors that influence the number of calories expended during aerobic performance: duration (how long you train) and intensity (how hard you train). For any given level of calories burned, these factors display an inverse relationship: If you train harder, then you don't have to train as long; if you train longer, then you don't have to train as hard.

In addition to an increase in energy expenditure while exercising, cardio also affects a phenomenon called excess postexercise oxygen consumption (EPOC). EPOC is a measure of the energy expended after a workout to return your body to its resting state. Factors contributing to this afterburn include replenishing glycogen stores, clearing lactic acid, reoxygenating blood, restoring hormonal levels, reestablishing normal core temperature, and synthesizing proteins for tissue remodeling. Importantly, EPOC is positively correlated with aerobic intensity: Higher intensities of training are associated with a greater postexercise afterburn.

The fat-burning benefits don't stop there.

Cardio also results in a number of chronic adaptations that promote fat loss. For one, it increases circulatory capacity. To be used as an energy source, fat must first enter the bloodstream for transport to target tissues. The thing is, blood flow tends to be poor in fatty regions, making it difficult to mobilize from these areas. The more capillaries you have, the easier it is for your body to liberate fat from stubborn areas so that it can use it as fuel. Also, your mitochondria (cellular furnaces where fat burning takes place) expand in size and number, and your aerobic enzymes (chemical messengers that accelerate the fat-burning process) increase in quantity. On top of all that, there's a sensitizing effect on insulin function, facilitating a greater capacity to store carbohydrate as glycogen rather than as fat.

In addition to having a positive effect on fat loss, cardio also enhances your ability to recuperate from intense resistance training. The increased capillarization associated with regular aerobic training facilitates nutrient exchange, providing your muscles with the substances required for repair and growth. Moreover, cardio serves as a form of active recovery. Blood is shunted to the working muscles during aerobic activity, further enhancing nutrient delivery and the removal of metabolic byproducts. It's why muscle stiffness and inflammation are alleviated by performing a bout of cardio.

Given all of these beneficial effects, it would seem like a no-brainer to include cardio as part of your overall training program, right?

Not so fast . . .

There's a potential downside to performing cardio in combination with intense lifting—a practice called concurrent training. The issue is that aerobic exercise and resistance exercise have opposing effects on cell signaling. Some researchers have compared the process to a switch whereby aerobic endurance exercise activates catabolic signaling and lifting weights activates anabolic signaling. The evidence suggests that the concept of a switch is overly simplistic; intracellular signaling is a highly complex phenomenon, and both anabolic and catabolic stimuli occur during most types of exercise. Still, there is some credence to the concept that catabolic processes predominate in aerobic training; thus, concurrent exercise has the potential to interfere with muscle development. This has led to the chronic interference hypothesis, which postulates that muscle cannot simultaneously adapt to the demands of concurrent training. Consistent with the chronic interference hypothesis, a recent meta-analysis found that muscular gains were significantly greater in those who solely lifted weights than in those who combined resistance training with cardio (Wilson et al., 2012).

The negative effects of cardio on muscle development may extend beyond interfering with cell signaling. Namely, people have upper limits as to how much exercise they can endure before becoming overtrained. Each cardio session adds to the total amount of training-related stress placed on your body. Beyond a certain point, the cumulative stresses of exercise will overtax your recuperative capacity. Over time, you'll wind up overtrained, further compromising muscle development.

So, should you include cardio in your routine? The answer is an unqualified yes! If nothing else, cardio provides a wide array of health benefits. Your heart, brain, lungs, blood vessels, and virtually every other part of your body will derive positive effects. So even if you aren't concerned with "leaning out," performing some cardio on a regular basis is a good idea.

If you desire body fat loss, adding extra cardio to the mix can enhance your results. The key is to balance the amount of cardio performed so that it doesn't negatively affect muscle. Following are some guidelines to help you achieve this balance to optimize your body composition.

CARDIO PROGRAMMING

Recall that duration and intensity are the primary cardio-related factors involved in fat burning and that an inverse relationship exists between these variables; namely, longer durations of low-intensity cardio are required to burn an equivalent number of calories as higher-intensity cardio performed for shorter durations. Two basic strategies exist to carry out cardio programming within this framework: low-intensity steady-state (LISS) exercise and high-intensity interval training (HIIT).

LISS involves exercising continuously at a pace below your lactate threshold—the point at which lactic acid rapidly accumulates in the bloodstream. Intensity during LISS can vary from very easy to somewhat hard. A leisurely walk and a jog would constitute the opposite ends of this spectrum. Again, because a jog expends more energy per minute than a walk, you'd have to spend more time walking to burn a similar number of calories as you would jogging. A simple way to determine LISS intensity is via the talk test, as discussed in chapter 6. To review, if you can carry on a conversation while training, then you are below your lactate threshold; if your speech pattern becomes labored so that sentences are disjointed, then you're training too hard for LISS. A rating of perceived exercise (RPE) scale can also be used to gauge intensity (see table 11.1). An RPE of about 4 to 6 would be appropriate for a low- to moderate-intensity steady-state workout.

HIIT takes aerobic training to another level. In its basic form, HIIT involves alternating between high-intensity and low-intensity periods of cardio. During high-intensity intervals, you train at a level above your lactate threshold, whereas during low-intensity intervals you train at a leisurely pace so that your body has time to clear lactic acid and replenish energy capacity.

Without question, HIIT accomplishes fat burning more efficiently than steady-state cardio does. Depending on the specifics of the respective protocols, you can burn approximately the same number of calories performing a HIIT routine in less than half the time as a LISS routine. If you're one of those people who would rather undergo dental surgery than engage in an extended cardio session, this is a big plus.

An emerging body of research indicates that HIIT can be a more effective fat burner than LISS from an absolute standpoint (Schoenfeld & Dawes, 2009). Some researchers have attributed the fat-burning advantage to an increase in EPOC. On a superficial level, there is validity to this hypothesis. Recall that EPOC is intensity dependent. There simply isn't much disturbance of homeostasis when cardio is performed at a low intensity of effort. As such, the afterburn from a bout of LISS lasts only a couple of hours, amounting to a few dozen extra calories expended—certainly nothing to get excited about. Alternatively, EPOC following a HIIT session can keep metabolism elevated for a half day or more, resulting in a substantially greater energy cost.

Here's the rub: Studies on the topic have not accounted for the effects of concurrent resistance training. Lifting weights has a much greater effect on EPOC than even the highest-intensity cardio bout. It is estimated that the afterburn

Table 11.1 RPE Scale

RPE	Intensity
1	Rest
2	Minimal exertion
3	Just above minimal exertion
4	Light exertion
5	Moderate exertion
6	Somewhat difficult
7	Difficult
8	Very difficult
9	Extremely difficult
10	Maximum effort

following a lifting session lasts for up to 72 hours, resulting in as much as 300 additional calories burned! This appears to be largely due to the increased protein synthesis needed for repairing and regenerating muscle tissue. What isn't clear is whether performing HIIT would add to the afterburn of a lifting session or simply be redundant. Although no research has been done on the topic, logic suggests that any additional energy expenditure would be relatively modest. So, any fat-burning advantage of HIIT very well might disappear in those who lift intensely.

Considering the facts, which approach is best?

Ultimately, both LISS and HIIT can be effective options. There is some evidence that HIIT may have less of an interference effect than steady-state exercise does (Wilson et al., 2012), but this is likely a function of manipulating intensity and duration to account for individual recovery abilities. Some have even made the case that HIIT enhances muscle hypertrophy, but this appears to be specific to newbies for whom such training imposes an overload stimulus on muscles. In the end it really comes down to preference. Some like the convenience of HIIT, whereas others prefer a more leisurely pace to their cardio. It's ultimately up to you.

Regardless of which approach you choose, the potential for chronic interference underscores the importance of limiting duration or intensity (or both) to ensure the preservation of lean body mass. I tend to err on the side of caution here. I've seen the best results from keeping the amount of cardio fairly low and manipulating nutritional intake to achieve optimal reductions in body fat.

The specifics of your program will depend on such factors as your recovery ability, the type and duration of your aerobic training, and your training experience. That said, here are some basic recommendations to guide your initial cardio efforts. If you prefer LISS, it can be performed four to six days a week at a

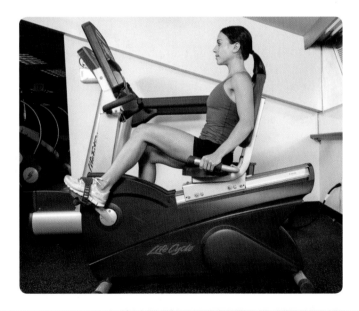

Experiment with different cardio approaches and determine what works best for you.

low to moderate intensity for about 30 to 45 minutes per session. A typical HIIT routine should last 20 to 30 minutes and be performed on three nonconsecutive days a week using a 1:1 high-to-low ratio (usually one-minute bouts for each interval segment). Again, these guidelines should be tailored to your needs and abilities. You also can combine approaches performing HIIT on some days and LISS on alternate days. Experiment with these approaches and determine what works best for you.

Understand that the number of calories burned in each cardio bout will be rather modest. A typical session will burn a few hundred calories. Although this certainly will help with weight control, it's not going to get you shredded. You can, of course, bump up caloric expenditure by upping the intensity or duration, or both. Unfortunately, this also increases the risk of compromising muscular development. Only you can decide whether this is a worthy trade-off. Assess your progress over time, paying special heed to any symptoms of overtraining, and adjust intensity and duration accordingly.

CHOOSING A MODALITY

Probably the question most often asked about cardio is, What aerobic activity burns the most calories? In actuality, there is no best cardiorespiratory exercise. It all comes down to duration and intensity: If you perform two activities of similar duration and intensity, you will achieve similar results in terms of calories burned (there will be some variances based on genetic factors, but their overall effect is relatively minor).

Your best approach is to choose exercises that you like doing. If you enjoy an activity, you'll be more likely to stick with it over the long haul. That said, I

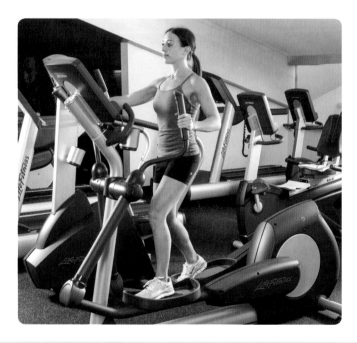

Select a cardio modality based on preference.

encourage you to keep an open mind and experiment with as many activities as possible; sometimes you'll enjoy an exercise more as time goes on. Variety tends to help people maintain interest and thus boost adherence.

With respect to cardio, variety is referred to as cross-training. Cross-training can be accomplished by performing as few as two activities (although more is certainly fine) and alternating them from one workout to the next. Not only does this keep your training routine from getting stale, but it also reduces the likelihood of a training-related injury. Because modalities use different muscles, your bones, muscles, and joints aren't subjected to continual impact. There is less wear and tear on your body, saving your musculoskeletal system from overuse.

Interestingly, running seems to negatively affect muscle adaptations more than other cardio modalities. It's believed that the associated high ground reaction forces combined with accentuated eccentric actions cause excessive muscle damage that inhibits recuperative abilities and thus blunts muscle development. The detrimental effects of running appear to be especially pronounced when you're in a caloric deficit and thus more prone to overtraining. Now, this doesn't mean that you shouldn't run. But if you do, limit the number of sessions per week, and cross-train with modalities that minimize ground reaction forces such as cycling and elliptical training.

Fasted or Fed?

A popular fat loss strategy involves performing cardio after an overnight fast. The rationale for the strategy is based on research showing that low glycogen levels cause your body to shift substrate use away from carbohydrate, thereby allowing greater mobilization of stored fat for energy. Many physique athletes swear by the practice, claiming that it's the key to a truly lean physique.

Although the theory that fasted cardio is superior for fat loss is certainly intriguing, it is based on an extrapolation of findings that might not translate into practice. A recent study from my lab indicates that training fasted might not be all that it's cracked up to be from a fat loss standpoint (Schoenfeld, Aragon, et al., 2014). We put a group of college-aged women on a strict diet and had them perform an hour of steady-state cardio three days per week. One group of subjects was given a meal immediately before the cardio bouts; another group was given the same meal immediately afterward. After four weeks, both groups had lost a significant amount of weight and fat mass, but there were no differences in body composition changes between the two groups.

What the study shows is that you can't simply look at fat burning in isolation. It really doesn't make a difference how much fat you burn during an exercise bout. What matters is the total amount of fat burned over the course of days and weeks. Understand that your body constantly adjusts its fuel use. If more fat is used for energy at one point, the body generally compensates by using more carbohydrate later on—and vice versa. In support of this fact, eating prior to cardio has been shown to increase a phenomenon called the thermic effect of exercise. In simple terms, this means that a preexercise meal enhances fat burning after the bout, and the effects persist for as much as 24 hours postworkout.

So does this mean that there is no benefit to performing fasted cardio?

Not necessarily.

It has been speculated that the true benefit of fasted cardio is specific to those with low levels of body fat (for a woman that would equate to less than about 15 percent) who are trying to lose that last bit of stubborn fat. Whether this outcome plays out in practice is yet to be determined.

What I can say with a high degree of confidence is that if fasted cardio does increase fat burning (still highly equivocal), the overall impact would be minor at best. ➡

Although the strategy might be advantageous to those who are very lean, performing exercise before a morning meal could just as easily have a negative impact on fat burning as a result of a decreased thermic effect of eating. All things considered, the best advice here would be to experiment with both strategies and determine what works best for you. It shouldn't make much of a difference either way in the end, so personal preference should be the final determinant.

Appendix

WORKOUT LOG

Date: _____   Body weight: _____
Time started: _____   Body fat percent: _____
Time finished: _____   Workout rating: _____

Strength Training Workout

Exercise	Set 1 Weight/reps	Set 2 Weight/reps	Set 3 Weight/reps	Set 4 Weight/reps	Set 5 Weight/reps

Strength training notes: _____
_____
_____

Cardio Workout

Exercise	Level	Time	Distance

Cardio notes: _____
_____
Other notes: _____
_____

From B. Schoenfeld, 2016, *Strong & sculpted* (Champaign, IL: Human Kinetics).

References

Carregaro, R., Cunha, R., Oliveira, C.G., Brown, L.E., & Bottaro, M. (2013). Muscle fatigue and metabolic responses following three different antagonist pre-load resistance exercises. *Journal of Electromyography and Kinesiology, 23* (5), 1090-1096. doi:10.1016/j.jelekin.2013.04.010

Fiatarone, M.A., Marks, E.C., Ryan, N.D., Meredith, C.N., Lipsitz, L.A., & Evans, W.J. (1990). High-intensity strength training in nonagenarians: Effects on skeletal muscle. *JAMA: The Journal of the American Medical Association, 263* (22), 3029-3034.

Fry, A.C., & Kraemer, W.J. (1997). Resistance exercise overtraining and overreaching: Neuroendocrine responses. *Sports Medicine* (Auckland, NZ), *23* (2), 106-129.

Gentil, P., Soares, S.R., Pereira, M.C., Cunha, R.R., Martorelli, S.S., Martorelli, A.S., & Bottaro, M. (2013). Effect of adding single-joint exercises to a multi-joint exercise resistance-training program on strength and hypertrophy in untrained subjects. *Applied Physiology, Nutrition, and Metabolism, 38* (3), 341-344. doi:10.1139/apnm-2012-0176

Hackett D.A., Johnson, N.A., Halaki, M., Chow, C.M. (2012). A novel scale to assess resistance-exercise effort. *J Sports Sci,* 30(13):1405-1413.

Henschke, N., & Lin, C.C. (2011). Stretching before or after exercise does not reduce delayed-onset muscle soreness. *British Journal of Sports Medicine, 45* (15), 1249-1250. doi:10.1136/bjsports-2011-090599

Izquierdo, M., Ibañez, J., González-Badillo, J.J., Häkkinen, K., Ratamess, N.A., Kraemer, W.J., French, D.N., Eslava, J., Altadill, A., Asiain, X., Gorostiaga, E.M. (2006). Differential effects of strength training leading to failure versus not to failure on hormonal responses, strength, and muscle power gains. *Journal of Applied Physiology* (Bethesda, MD, 1985), *100* (5), 1647-1656. doi:10.1152/japplphysiol.01400.2005

Krieger, J.W. (2009). Single versus multiple sets of resistance exercise: A meta-regression. *Journal of Strength and Conditioning Research, 23* (6), 1890-1901. doi:10.1519/JSC.0b013e3181b370be

Krieger, J.W. (2010). Single vs. multiple sets of resistance exercise for muscle hypertrophy: A meta-analysis. *Journal of Strength and Conditioning Research, 24* (4), 1150-1159. doi:10.1519/JSC.0b013e3181d4d436

Morton, S.K., Whitehead, J.R., Brinkert, R.H., & Caine, D.J. (2011). Resistance training vs. static stretching: Effects on flexibility and strength. *Journal of Strength and Conditioning Research, 25* (12), 3391-3398. doi:10.1519/JSC.0b013e31821624aa

Ogborn, D., & Schoenfeld, B.J. (2014). The role of fiber types in muscle hypertrophy: Implications for loading strategies. *Strength & Conditioning Journal, 36* (2), 20-25.

Ribeiro, A.S., Romanzini, M., Schoenfeld, B.J., Souza, M.F., Avelar, A., & Cyrino, E.S. (2014). Effect of different warm-up procedures on the performance of resistance training exercises. *Perceptual and Motor Skills, 119* (1), 133-145. doi:10.2466/25.29.PMS.119c17z7

Schoenfeld, B.J., Aragon, A.A., Wilborn, C.D., Krieger, J.W., & Sonmez, G.T. (2014). Body composition changes associated with fasted versus non-fasted aerobic exercise. *Journal of the International Society of Sports Nutrition, 11* (1), 54-014-0054-7. eCollection 2014. doi:10.1186/s12970-014-0054-7

Schoenfeld, B.J., Contreras, B., Tiryaki-Sonmez, G., Wilson, J.M., Kolber, M.J., & Peterson, M.D. (2015). Regional differences in muscle activation during hamstrings exercise. *Journal of Strength and Conditioning Research, 29* (1), 159-164. doi:10.1519/JSC.0000000000000598

Schoenfeld, B., & Dawes, J. (2009). High-intensity interval training: Applications for general fitness training. *Strength & Conditioning Journal, 31* (6), 44-46.

Schoenfeld, B.J., Peterson, M.D., Ogborn, D., Contreras, B., & Sonmez, G.T. (2015). Effects of low- versus high-load resistance training on muscle strength and hypertrophy in well-trained men. *Journal of Strength and Conditioning Research,* 29(10):2954-63

Schoenfeld, B.J., Wilson, J.M., Lowery, R.P., & Krieger, J.W. (2014). Muscular adaptations in low- versus high-load resistance training: A meta-analysis. *European Journal of Sport Science,* 1-10. doi:10.1080/17461391.2014.989922

Thacker, S.B., Gilchrist, J., Stroup, D.F., & Kimsey, C.D., Jr. (2004). The impact of stretching on sports injury risk: A systematic review of the literature. *Medicine & Science in Sports & Exercise, 36* (3), 371-378. doi:00005768-200403000-00004 [pii]

Wakahara, T., Fukutani, A., Kawakami, Y., & Yanai, T. (2013). Nonuniform muscle hypertrophy: Its relation to muscle activation in training session. *Medicine & Science in Sports & Exercise, 45* (11), 2158-2165. doi:10.1249/MSS.0b013e3182995349; 10.1249/MSS.0b013e3182995349

Wakahara, T., Miyamoto, N., Sugisaki, N., Murata, K., Kanehisa, H., Kawakami, Y., Fukunaga, T., Yanai, T. (2012). Association between regional differences in muscle activation in one session of resistance exercise and in muscle hypertrophy after resistance training. *European Journal of Applied Physiology, 112* (4), 1569-1576. doi:10.1007/s00421-011-2121-y

Wilson, J.M., Marin, P.J., Rhea, M.R., Wilson, S.M., Loenneke, J.P., & Anderson, J.C. (2012). Concurrent training: A meta-analysis examining interference of aerobic and resistance exercises. *Journal of Strength and Conditioning Research, 26* (8), 2293-2307. doi:10.1519/JSC.0b013e31823a3e2d

Index

Note: Page references followed by an italicized *f* or *t* indicate information contained in figures and tables, respectively.

About the Author

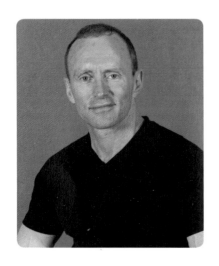

Brad Schoenfeld, PhD, CSCS, CSPS, FNSCA, is an internationally renowned fitness expert and widely regarded as one of the leading authorities on body composition training. He is the author of several fitness books, including Women's Home Workout Bible (Human Kinetics, 2010), Sculpting Her Body Perfect (Human Kinetics, 2008), 28-Day Body Shapeover (Human Kinetics, 2006), and Look Great Naked (Prentice Hall, 2001).

Schoenfeld has been published or appeared in numerous publications including *Shape, Self, Fitness, Oxygen, Muscle and Fitness Hers, Women's Health, Prevention, Ladies Home Journal, Redbook, Cosmopolitan, Marie Claire, Woman's Day, New York Times, New York Daily News, Gannett Suburban Papers, Washington Post, Chicago Tribune, Men's Health,* and *Ironman.* He is a regular contributor to several magazines, including *FitnessRx,* and serves as a fitness expert and writer for popular websites including Bodybuilding.com and T-Nation.com. He has been a fitness correspondent for *News 12* in Westchester, New York, and has appeared on more than 100 television shows and networks, including *CBS Evening News, CNN Headline News, Fox News, UPN News, Good Day New York, Good Day LA, CBS New York Live, NBC Live at Five,* and *Today in New York,* as well as hundreds of radio programs across the United States.

Schoenfeld is a consultant to Reebok International and provides educational content for their ReebokOne program. He also is on the advisory board for Dymatize Nutrition, a leading manufacturer of nutritional supplements. He was formerly the national spokesperson for Dreamfields Foods, makers of the world's premier low-carb pasta.

Schoenfeld's speaking credits include seminars for the International Health, Racquet and Sportsclub Association (IHRSA); National Strength and Conditioning Association (NSCA); American College of Sports Medicine (ACSM); ECA World Fitness; CanFitPro; Athletic Business Conference; and Club Industry.

Schoenfeld earned his PhD in health science at Rocky Mountain University while researching the mechanisms of muscle hypertrophy and their application to resistance training. He has authored more than 80 peer-reviewed scientific articles. He is a certified strength and conditioning specialist with the NSCA. He was named NSCA Personal Trainer of the Year in 2011 and elected to the NSCA Board of Directors in 2012. He has achieved multiple certifications as a personal trainer from the NSCA, ACSM, American Council on Exercise, Aerobics and Fitness Association of America, and CanFitPro. He is a member of IDEA Health and Fitness Association, which has bestowed on him the title of master trainer, the highest ranking possible.